Medication Safety

Medication Safety

An Essential Guide

Edited by

Molly Courtenay and Matt Griffiths

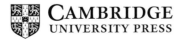

CAMBRIDGE
UNIVERSITY PRESS

CAMBRIDGE UNIVERSITY PRESS
Cambridge, New York, Melbourne, Madrid, Cape Town, Singapore,
São Paulo, Delhi, Dubai, Tokyo

Cambridge University Press
The Edinburgh Building, Cambridge CB2 8RU, UK

Published in the United States of America by
Cambridge University Press, New York

www.cambridge.org
Information on this title:
www.cambridge.org/9780521721639

First published 2010

Printed in the United Kingdom at the University Press, Cambridge

*A catalogue record for this publication is available from the
British Library*

ISBN 978-0-521-72163-9 Paperback

Contents

Contributors

Alison Blenkinsopp
Professor of the Practice of Pharmacy, School of Pharmacy, Keele University, Staffordshire, UK

Molly Courtenay
Division of Health and Social Care, Faculty of Health and Medical Sciences, The University of Surrey

Gill Dorer
Honorary Research Fellow, University of Leeds School of Healthcare, Faculty of Medicine and Health, Leeds, UK

Martin Duerden
Consultant in Medicines Policy and Use, and Honorary Senior Lecturer, University College London, London, UK

Alison G. Eggleton
Principal Pharmacist, Education and Training, Cambridge University Hospitals NHS Foundation Trust, Cambridge, UK

Matt Griffiths
Senior Nurse, Medicines Management, University Hospitals of Leicester, and Visiting Professor of Prescribing and Medicines Management, School of Health, University of Northampton, Northampton, UK

Tim House
Medicines Information Manager, Medicines Information, Inpatient Safety, Addenbrooke's Hospital, Cambridge, UK

Rebecca Jester
Head of School of Nursing and Midwifery, Keele University, Staffordshire, UK

Roger Knaggs
Specialist Pharmacist, Anaesthesia and Pain Management, Nottingham University Hospitals NHS Trust, Nottingham, UK

Simon de Lusignan
Chair, Primary Care Informatics Working Group of the European Federation for Medical Informatics (EFMI)

Liz Plastow
Independent Consultant for Nursing & Medicines Management, Specialist Community Public Health Nursing, Wilmington, Honiton, Devon, UK

Imogen Savage
Senior Lecturer in Patient Safety, The School of Pharmacy, University of London, London, UK

Sharon Smart
Clinical Director, SCHIN Ltd, Newcastle Upon Tyne, UK

Jasmeet Soar
Consultant in Anaesthetics & Intensive Care Medicine, North Bristol NHS Trust, Southmead Hospital, Bristol, UK

Jon Standing
Senior Pharmacist, Medicines Information Manager, Medicines Information, Pharmacy Department, Southmead Hospital, Bristol, UK

Anne Twidell
Merrow, Guildford, Surrey, UK

Jane Wastson
Medicines Management Lead, Tiverton, Devon, UK

Sheena Williamson
Senior Lecturer, University of Stirling, Department of Nursing and Midwifery, Centre for Health Science, Inverness, UK

Preface

Non-medical prescribing is a new area of practice for nurses, pharmacists and allied health professionals (AHPS). Over 30 000 district nurses and health visitors are able to prescribe from the Nurse Prescribers Formulary (NPF) for Community Practitioners. More than 14 000 nurses and 1500 pharmacists across the United Kingdom (UK) have virtually the same independent prescribing rights as doctors. Several hundred AHPs (i.e. physiotherapists, podiatrists, chiropodists and radiologists) and optometrists are able to prescribe in partnership with doctors. These figures are set to rise.

Errors surrounding the prescription, administration and dispensing of medicines by healthcare professionals account for a significant amount of harm and even deaths across the UK. Twenty per cent of all critical incidents in the National Health Service (NHS) are caused by medication errors. These errors cost the NHS as much as it would cost to fund two acute teaching hospitals. The reduction of prescribing errors is now a major Government initiative. This timely and much needed text is designed for all healthcare professionals involved in the management of medicines.

Chapter 1, introduction, provides a general overview of medication safety, the different mechanisms available to healthcare professionals to deliver medicines to patients and actions that can be taken to improve medication safety. Chapters 2 to 4 examine safety in prescribing, safety in dispensing and safety in administering. Adverse drug reactions and drug interactions, interface of care and communication and parenteral drug administration, are explored in Chapters 5 to 7. Chapters 8 to 10 deal with calculations, controlled drugs and patient safety, reporting medication incidents and near misses. The final chapter, Chapter 11, focuses on ensuring safety through evidence-based medicine.

Each chapter is fully referenced and, where appropriate, readers are offered suggestions for further reading and other information sources. We hope that that this book will make a positive contribution to a very important aspect of patient care.

Molly Courtenay
Matt Griffiths

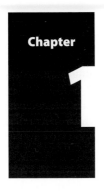

Chapter 1

Introduction to medication errors and medication safety

Molly Courtenay and Matt Griffiths

A medication safety incident is defined by the National Patient Safety Agency (NPSA) as:

'any unintended or unexpected incident which could have or did lead to harm for one or more patients' (NPSA, 2007:9).

These incidents can occur at each stage of the process involved in the delivery of medicines to patients, i.e. prescribing (including transcribing or physician ordering), dispensing, preparation, administering and monitoring (NPSA, 2007). Medication incidents have been reported as accounting for 10%–20% of all Adverse Events (AE) (Department of Health (DoH), 2004), i.e. an event that causes an unintended injury to a patient that either prolongs hospitalization or produces disability (Karson & Bates, 1999).

The impact of medication safety incidents on patient outcomes includes increased length of stay, disability and mortality (Vincent *et al.*, 2001). Across the UK, about two and a half million medicines are prescribed across hospitals and the community every day (DoH, 2004) and an indicator of quality, adopted to demonstrate medication safety, is the incidence of medication errors (DoH, 2004). The Government has committed to reducing the incidents of medication errors in prescribed drugs by 40% (DoH, 2004).

Between January 2005 and June 2006, 60 000 medication incidents were reported to the NPSA via the National Reporting and Learning System (NRLS) (NPSA, 2007). Although most medicine-related activity is carried out in the community, over 80% of the incidents reported to the NPSA were from the hospital setting. The majority of these incidents (over 80%) did not result in harm. Wrong dose, strength or frequency of medicine, omitted medicine and wrong medicine were errors that occurred most frequently and accounted for nearly 60% of all incidents reported.

Ninety-two out of the 60 000 medication incidents reported to the NPSA resulted in severe harm or death and arose from errors involving the administration and prescribing of medicines. Medicines most frequently associated with these incidents included opioids, anticoagulants, anaesthetics, insulin, antibiotics, chemotherapy, anti-psychotics and infusion fluids. The two groups of patients associated with medication errors, and highlighted in the NPSA report, included patients with known allergies being given medicines to which they were allergic (notably antibiotics), and errors involving specific medicines and dose calculations in children up to 4 years old.

Other important areas highlighted by the report included the high number of injectable medicines resulting in death and severe harm; risks associated with care transfer and the importance of accurate documentation; the availability and supply of certain medicines at the point they are required; medicines given outside a medicines ward round, or to those patients with specific needs.

Medication Safety: An Essential Guide, ed. Molly Courtenay and Matt Griffiths. Published by Cambridge University Press. © M. Courtenay and M. Griffiths 2009.

Legislative changes over the last decade mean that there are now a number of groups of healthcare professionals, in addition to doctors, able to prescribe medicines for patients. As of 1994, community nurse practitioners have been able independently to prescribe from a limited list of medicines. Independent prescribing rights were later extended in 2001 to include any appropriately qualified first level registered nurse and, as of 2006, Nurse Independent Prescribers (NIPs) have been able independently to prescribe any licensed medicine for any condition and some controlled drugs (CDs) provided that it is within their area of competence (DoH, 2005). These nurses are also able to prescribe any medicine as a supplementary prescriber (DoH, 2002), i.e. prescribe any medicine for any condition in partnership with a doctor and provided that the medicine is within their area of competence and listed on the patient's Clinical Management Plan (CMP).

As of 2003 (DoH, 2002), appropriately qualified pharmacists have been able to prescribe any medicine as a supplementary prescriber. In 2006 legislative changes (DoH, 2005) enabled these healthcare professionals independently to prescribe any licensed medicine (apart from controlled drugs).

In 2005, legislative changes enabled the prescription of medicine by optometrists and allied health professionals (i.e. physiotherapists, radiographers, and chiropodists/podiatrists) under supplementary prescribing. Further changes to legislation in 2007 (DoH, 2007) enabled appropriately qualified optometrists to independently prescribe any licensed medicine for ocular conditions affecting the eye, and the tissues surrounding the eye, within the recognized area of expertise and competence of the optometrist.

There are now approximately 14 000 nurses, 1500 pharmacists, and several hundred optometrists and AHPs able to prescribe medicines and these numbers are set to rise. The latest figures from the NHS Information Centre (http://www.ic.nhs.uk/) show that in the year ending March 2008, nurses in primary care prescribed items worth £29.2 m. In the year ending March 2009, this figure was £33.0 m i.e. a percentage increase of 13.1%. Pharmacists prescribed items worth £205 000 up to year end March 2008 and £381 000 up to March 2009 i.e. a percentage increase of 86.0%. The figure for GP prescribing for 2008 (January-December) was £7.9 billion.

Training for non-medical prescribers involves 27 days in the classroom (although some programmes have a distance learning element) and 12 days in practice with a Designated Medical Practitioner (DMP) responsible for the education and assessment of the prescribing student. A range of techniques are used to assess students' prescribing knowledge (which includes assessment of numeracy and drug calculation skills). In response to increasing numbers of nurses being involved in the prescription of medicines for children, it is now a requirement that nurse prescribers are competent to prescribe for children, or know when to refer to another prescriber when working outside their area of clinical competence (Nursing and Midwifery Council (NMC), 2008).

In addition to the expansion of prescribing rights to these groups of healthcare professionals, exemptions in the Medicines Act enable paramedics and midwives to supply or administer medicines, and a number of different groups of healthcare professionals (including midwives, nurses, pharmacists, optometrists, podiatrists/chiropodists, radiographers, orthoptists, physiotherapists, and ambulance paramedics) are also able to supply or administer medicines to patients under Patient Group Directions (PGDs). A PGD, signed by a doctor and agreed by a pharmacist, acts as a direction to supply and/ or administer a Prescription Only Medicine (POM) to a patient (using their own assessment of patient need) without necessarily referring back to a doctor for an individual prescription. PGDs 'fit' best in services where the use of medicines follows a predictable pattern and are less individualized (National Prescribing Centre (NPC), 2004). The use of PGDs are popular, for example, in first contact services where one-off treatments are required as opposed to a number of treatments over a long period of time.

It is evident that around 90% of the 14 000 Nurse Independent/Nurse Supplementary Prescribers are prescribing medicines (Courtenay & Carey, 2008a). Although the majority of these nurses are in primary care, increasing numbers of nurses from secondary care are accessing the prescribing programme. Nearly a third of these nurses prescribe medicines for diabetic patients and nearly 50% of these nurses prescribe insulins (Courtenay & Carey, 2008b, c). Although there are currently restrictions surrounding the prescription of CDs, there is some evidence that lifting these restrictions in the area of acute and chronic pain in the hospital setting will increase the prescription of these medicines (Stenner & Courtenay, 2007). Proposals to lift these restrictions are currently awaited (Home Office (HO), 2007). Several researchers have identified factors that may lead to errors with regards to the prescription of medicines by non-medical prescribers. These factors include a lack of questioning by nurses about allergies to medicines (Latter *et al.*, 2005), a lack of access to patient records (Candlish *et al.*, 2006; Hall *et al.*, 2006), duplication of records and transcription errors (Bradley & Nolan, 2007; Weiss *et al.*, 2006). Insulin and opioids were medicines associated most frequently with incidences reported to the NPSA that resulted in severe harm or death. Patients with known allergies being given medicines to which they were allergic, risks associated with care transfer and the importance of accurate documentation were all areas highlighted by the report.

The NPSA have identified seven key actions to improve medication safety. These actions include:

- Increased reporting and learning from medication incidents.
- Implementation by NPSA of safer medication practice recommendations.
- Improved staff skills and competence.
- Minimization of dosing errors.
- Ensurance that medicines are not omitted.
- Ensurance that correct medicines are given to the correct patient.
- Documentation of patients' allergy status.

These actions apply to all healthcare professionals involved in delivering medicines to patients, including those on undergraduate programmes. Additionally, given the recent legislative changes expanding prescribing powers to include other groups of healthcare professionals (in addition to doctors) and the research evidence described above, it would seem particularly important that those responsible for the education and training of non-medical prescribers are aware of these actions.

The lack of incidents reported in the community to the NPSA perhaps highlights the need to monitor patients in these settings more closely – particularly as the majority of nurse prescribers work in primary care settings. One way to encourage such reporting would be to make the reporting of errors a statutory requirement as opposed to a professional one.

Other schemes and initiatives that would help to ensure medicine safety, some of which are simple and others that would require a substantial investment, include:

The red tabard scheme, ensuring nurses undertaking medication rounds are not disturbed.

Specifically designed intravenous (IV) connectors, that only allow attachment of IV syringes.

Specifically designed naso-gastric tubes that do not enable the attachment of IV syringes.

Specific medicine labels that can be transferred to IV syringes.

Allergy bands for patients with known allergies.

Medication administration charts that clearly identify those patients with allergies on each page of the chart.

Bar coding of both medicines and patients' identity bracelets to ensure medicines are given to the correct patient.

Electronic prescribing.

Safe storage of medicines.

The NPSA estimates that preventable harm from medicines could cost England as much as £750 million each year. Statistically, we as individuals or our loved ones will almost certainly be victims of a medication error. The reduction of prescribing errors is now a major Government initiative (National Patient Safety Agency (NPSA), 2007). Given this initiative, combined with the recent introduction of non-medical prescribing, this is a timely and much needed text.

References

Bradley E, Nolan P. (2007). Impact of nurse prescribing: a qualitative study. *Journal of Advanced Nursing*, **59** (2),120–8.

Candlish CA, Puri A, Sackville MP. (2006). A survey of supplementary prescribing pharmacists from the Sunderland pharmacy school. *International Journal of Pharmaceutical Practice*, **14**, B42–3.

Courtenay M, Carey N. (2008a). Nurse Independent Prescribing and Nurse Supplementary Prescribing: National questionnaire survey. *Journal of Advanced Nursing*, **61** (3), 291–9.

Courtenay M, Carey NJ. (2008b). Preparing nurses to prescribe medicines for patients with diabetes: a national questionnaire survey. *Journal of Advanced Nursing*, **61**(4), 403–12.

Courtenay M, Carey NJ. (2008c). The prescribing practices of nurse independent prescribers caring for patients with diabetes. *Practical Diabetes International*, **25**(4), 152–7.

DoH (2004). *Building a safer NHS for patients: improving medication safety*: A report by the Chief Pharmaceutical Officer, London: Department of Health.

DoH (2002). *Supplementary Prescribing for Nurses and Pharmacists within the NHS in England*, London: Department of Health.

DoH (2005). *Written Ministerial Statement on the expansion of independent nurse prescribing and introduction of pharmacists independent prescribing*, London: Department of Health.

DoH (2007). *Optometrists to Get Independent Prescribing Rights (press release)*. London: Department of Health.

Hall J, Cantrill J, Noyce, P. (2006). Why don't trained community nurse prescribers prescribe? *Journal of Clinical Nursing*, **15**, 403–12.

HO (2007) Public Consultation – *Independent Prescribing of Controlled Drugs by Nurse and Pharmacist Independent Prescribers.* London: Home Office.

Karson AS, Bates DW. (1999). Screening for adverse events, *Journal of Evaluation in Clinical Practice*, **5**(1), 23–32.

Latter S, Maben J, Myall M, Courtenay M, Young A, Dunn N. (2005). *An evaluation of extended formulary independent nurse prescribing.* Final Report, Policy Research Programme Department of Health & University of Southampton NHS Business Services Authority (2007) http://www.ppa.nhs.uk/ppa/pres_vol_cost.htm.

NMC. Guidance for CPD for Nurse and Midwife Prescribers NMC circular 2008 10/2008.

NPC (2004). Patients group directions. *Liverpool*: NPC.

NPSA (2007). *Safety in doses: medication safety incident in the NHS: The fourth report from the Patient Safety Observatory.* London, NPSA.

Stenner K, Courtenay M. (2007). A qualitative study on the impact of legislation on prescribing of controlled drugs by nurses. *Nurse Prescribing*, **5**(6), 257–61.

Vincent C, Neale G, Woloshynowych M. (2001) Adverse events in British hospitals: preliminary retrospective record review, *British Medical Journal*, **322**, 517–19.

Weiss MC, Sutton J, Adams C. (2006). *Exploring Innovation in Pharmacy Practice: A Qualitative Evaluation of Supplementary Prescribing by Pharmacists.* London: Royal Pharmaceutical Society.

Safety in prescribing

Anne Twidell and Simon de Lusignan

Introduction

This chapter sets out the rationale for improving prescribing safety, namely the high rate of deaths, unnecessary hospital admissions and illness caused by unsafe prescribing; and what practical steps prescribers should take to reduce the risk of issuing an unsafe prescription. The tragedy in Northwick Park in 2006 when healthy volunteers suffered catastrophic consequences, albeit in the first test of a new drug, highlighted how pharmaceuticals need to be treated with caution and respect (Sunthralingham, 2006). However, it is not just new drugs which can be unsafe; drugs which have become established after many years of clinical use can also cause problems (Lasser *et al.*, 2002). For example, after several years of use, a widely used non-steroidal anti-inflammatory drug was found to be associated with an increased risk of myocardial infarction (Solomon *et al.*, 2004).

The first part of this chapter describes why prescribing safety is so important and this is addressed under the following four themes:

(1) **Key issues for safe prescribing at the point of care.** Theme one explores the safety issues that should be considered by an individual prescriber before issuing a prescription. A key message for prescribers is that they need to have the necessary information to hand at the point of prescribing: an understanding of the patient's wishes; access to a comprehensive medical record; and access to information about the drug they are about to prescribe.

(2) **Clinical governance and systems to ensure safe prescribing.** The second theme looks at the systems that should be in place to monitor and quality assure safe prescribing. Our key message here is that good prescribing must be in the context of ongoing audit and evaluation of its safety and effectiveness. Had systems been in place, including improved data quality on death certificates or indeed diamorphine use, the notorious Dr Harold Shipman may have been flagged as an outlier for his high death rate (Aylin *et al.*, 2004). The same principles may help identify unsafe practice of medicines.

(3) **Communication and team work.** Healthcare professionals increasingly work as part of multidisciplinary teams where effective communication is essential. Good communication with patients, including how to recognize and act on adverse events, and keeping good-quality records are essential.

(4) **Computer decision support systems and using technology to support safer prescribing.** Information technology (IT) has the potential to reduce prescribing errors. However, implementing IT systems in healthcare is challenging. IT is changing the nature of the clinical task from the clinician as the holder of information to having the skills to critically appraise the evidence. Patients and the

Medication Safety: An Essential Guide, ed. Molly Courtenay and Matt Griffiths. Published by Cambridge University Press. © M. Courtenay and M. Griffiths 2009.

public now have access to the same information as their prescriber (de Lusignan, 2003). This final theme explores these issues.

The chapter is written from the perspective of prescribers in the developed world, where the supply chains for pharmaceuticals and pharmacies are generally well regulated, safe and efficient. Issues relating to drug availability, cost, and risks associated with counterfeit medicines are beyond the scope of this chapter. Readers interested in these issues should explore the World Health Organization's (WHO) *Essential Drugs Programme* (WHO) and issues around the pharmacy supply chain and good pharmacy practice (International Pharmacy Federation). However, although the pharmacy supply chain is rarely an issue in developed countries, we do have some supply chain issues. These include:

Parallel imports. Parallel importing of medicines is the process of importing medications, due to be supplied to another country, at a lower cost. In the UK in the 1980s there were concerns surrounding the supply of these medications as their instructions for use were written in another language – potentially denying patients access to information which could impact on safety (Fullerton, 1984).

Generic substitution. Over the last two decades there has been a shift towards generic prescribing (i.e. prescribing by drug rather than brand name). However, generic equivalents may vary with regards to frequency of dose or application, and occasionally, this can affect bioavailability. Generic prescribing has rightly been driven as a cost-saving exercise in hard-pressed health services. Whilst a lot of data have been collected about bio-equivalence, few studies have explored the safety issues. An exception is the American Food and Drug Administration (FDA) which provides a searchable online database, which describes where generic substitution is or is not safe (Food and Drugs Administration). The authors' own experience is that some patients on long-term treatments may never be reassured that a generic medicine is equivalent to their branded alternative. Patients may prefer a particular brand (Mott & Cline, 2002). Prescribing the generic equivalent may actually put patients at risk because they are confused about a different physical appearance of one or more of their medications. In these situations it is more important that a patient takes their medicine, and so prescribing some by brand name is justified. Additionally, in some instances, the difference in bioavailability is sometimes clinically significant (Borgheini, 2003).

The remainder of the chapter examines prescribing errors, and the rate at which these errors occur. This is something that everyone involved in prescribing or health service management should be aware of, and actively take steps to reduce. No prescription is 100% safe, and decisions about prescribing should always take into account risk; modulated by patients' wishes. A key theme across this chapter is encouraging recognition of the complexity of prescribing decisions. We encourage prescribers to see their task as a complex, safety-critical decision.

Why is prescribing safety important?

Two landmark reports, both from the USA, identified high levels of medical error, of which prescribing errors comprised a major component. These two reports produced by the Institute of Medicine were called: *To Err is Human* (Committee on Quality of

Healthcare in America, 2000) and *Crossing the Quality Chasm* (Committee on Quality of Healthcare in America, 2001).

To Err is Human identified that 50–100 000 preventable errors result in death in the USA; that they are costly, and that systems can be improved and errors reduced. Probably the best known quote from *Crossing the Quality Chasm* is:

> '…between the health care that we now have, and the health care we could have, lies not just a gap, but a chasm.'

Although these reports addressed a wide range of issues about the importance of evidence-based patient-centred care, delivered in a timely, efficient and equitable way; they placed delivering safe healthcare at the top of its list. It is evident from these studies that as many as 10% of people admitted to hospital have had an adverse medical event, and that most of these events are prescribing errors (Committee on Quality of Healthcare in America, 2000). Prescribers in the UK have traditionally been medical practitioners; however, in recent years non-medical prescribers (nurses, pharmacists, radiographers, podiatrists, physiotherapists and optometrists) have become more prevalent. Although the majority of prescribing episodes are undertaken by medical prescribers, the number of non-medical prescribing episodes is increasing. To date, there have been no identified prescribing errors by non-medical prescribers in England. Unfortunately the profession of the prescriber in the National Reporting and Learning System (NRLS) dataset is not available (National Patients Safety Agency (NPSA), 2007). However, no prescriber can afford to be complacent; all need to be mindful of the potential hazards that can arise, and could apply to any prescribing professional.

Prescribing errors are embedded in current clinical practice. The rates of error remain high and there is a suggestion that not having sufficient time to think through all the relevant factors may be significant. Koppel *et al.* (2008) found that, where physicians cancel computer requested prescriptions, soon after placing an order, it is associated with prescribing errors. Where prescriptions are cancelled within 45 minutes, two-thirds of them are inappropriate – incorrect dose, etc. Where they are cancelled within 2 hours, 55% are inappropriate. One possible interpretation of these data is that information that led to the cancellation was not considered properly at the time of the prescription (Koppel *et al.*, 2008). It is known that neonatal prescribing errors can be dangerous and have severe consequences. Recent findings from a neonatal intensive care unit suggested that a lack of awareness amongst staff of drug safety issues was common, and identified prescribing and drug administration errors as the commonest causes of error (Kunac & Reith, 2005). The rate of non-compliance with good prescribing practice in neonatal paediatrics has been reported as being evident in 40% of prescriptions; though training and provision of better information systems has substantially reduced this figure (Pallas *et al.*, 2008).

In primary care adverse drug reactions are also common, many are preventable and can cause harm including unnecessary hospital admission. A systematic review by Thomsen *et al.* (2007) suggested that 85% of the preventable adverse reactions were caused by a small number of types of therapy: cardiovascular drugs, analgesia and hypoglycaemic agents. Interestingly, of the people who had unnecessary admissions, nearly half (45%) were inadequately monitored (Thomsen *et al.*, 2007). In an international study undertaken in primary care (in Canada, Australia, England, the Netherlands, New Zealand and the

United States) over a 7-month data collection period, the error rates per month of practice were similar; GPs saw around one error per month. Thirty to 40% of these errors were serious, i.e. resulting in harm to patients. Six to 7% of errors were very serious and resulted in hospital admission or death (Rosser *et al.*, 2005).

Errors by individuals, systems which perpetuate unsafe practice, poor teamwork and under-developed information systems all contribute to a situation where there are unnecessary medication errors.

Key issues for safe prescribing at the point of care

Is prescribing the right decision?

The first question which any prescribers should ask themselves is whether a prescription is really indicated. This is, in one sense, an easy question and, in another, extremely challenging. In many scenarios there is a non-drug option, which does not risk side effects or patient safety. For example, the natural history of viral warts and verruccae is that they get better – albeit over a considerable time period; the same is true for many cases of tennis and golfer's elbow. Many patients are very happy to await natural cure rather than risk the side effects of treatment. Cryotherapy for warts can leave a hypopigmented halo which is much more noticeable when the skin is tanned. Steroid injections for tennis elbow can risk skin thinning and infection.

Lifestyle change can sometimes be a much safer and effective option. For example, some people can make a significant reduction in their cholesterol by changing their diet, and so avoid the risks of statins. Some obese people can control their diabetes effectively by change in diet, exercising more and losing weight.

All prescribing has risks and the prescriber has to weigh up the risk–benefit ratio for the patient; and be strongly influenced by the wishes of the patient. The risk–benefit ratio should be considered in the context of the long-term relationship with the patient as well as the pros and cons of the particular decision.

For example, a patient who had previously had pneumonia may be very frightened by their next respiratory infection. Whilst the clinician might not normally prescribe for them based on the symptoms alone – the circumstances might dictate that the small risk to patient safety in prescribing is justified by the potential damage to the clinician–patient relationship if they do not.

The 'delayed prescription' is a halfway house between not prescribing and prescribing and where there is a possibility that a prescription is not required. This is a useful approach where a patient does not currently have symptoms but might deteriorate. It reduces both the number of prescriptions dispensed and risks associated with prescribing. For example, a patient may have a minor deterioration in their asthma symptoms. There are many patients in these circumstances who can be advised to increase their current inhalers, and given a 'delayed prescription' for an oral steroid and antibiotic should their condition deteriorate. This is recommended by the National Institute for Health & Clinical Excellence (NICE, 2008). The practice of delayed prescriptions also has the potential to be beneficial in reducing actual antibiotic use, which could be a major benefit in the current climate of overuse of antibiotics and the associated risks to public health.

It is essential when the decision is made to issue a prescription to explore treatment options and patient choice and that the final choice is as a result of a shared decision-making process. Most patients are happy with 'usual practice' but the internet has made information as widely available to patients as to clinicians. Open honest discussion of benefits and risks are an essential part of safe practice. Treatment options should always include the choice of no treatment and an explanation of the natural history of the condition. Shared decision-making can be checked by asking the patient if they would mind summarizing back the key points about the next steps.

The patient should be able to give informed consent. Usually, consent is implied rather than explicit, in that the patient usually accepts the prescription from the clinician, then takes it to the pharmacist for it to be dispensed. However, there are special circumstances where others speak on behalf of the patient. Commonly, this happens at the beginning and end of life. Children and young people usually have a parent as their prime carer; the elderly, their spouse or other relative. Problems with patient safety can arise where the carer either refuses what the clinician feels is the best treatment or wants something outside of best practice. For example, there is no clear-cut diagnostic test for asthma in very young children. This may be the clinician's diagnosis and yet the child's parent may not want them to have asthma and is not keen to try an inhaler or other therapy. The clinician needs to discuss carefully the level of risk with the carer; and if there is any significant risk with other team members.

Ultimately, the prescriber is the patient's advocate and is there to give best advice and recommend appropriate therapy, in each given circumstance. Prescribing is only one of many options. Before going on to issue a prescription, the prescriber needs to ensure that the patient has the right diagnosis and that the prescription they issue is safe. These issues are explored in the next two sections.

Right diagnosis/rational basis for prescribing

Traditional approaches to diagnosis use deductive reasoning and, like most processes, are not completely reliable. Medical students and junior doctors arrive at a diagnosis through carefully taking a detailed and systematic history, followed by examination and investigations (blood tests, X-rays, etc.) – so-called 'clerking' a patient. The diagnosis is largely based on the history combined with examination and investigation findings. A combined process of looking for recognizable patterns of disease and elimination contribute to the final diagnosis. Some diagnoses are reliable and others much less so. For example, heart failure and chronic obstructive pulmonary disease are both diseases usually secondary to cigarette smoking (in the former case by causing ischaemic heart disease, and in the latter by damaging the airways). Both occur in older people and often present with shortness of breath. Unfortunately, there is often clinical overlap between the two, and consequent inappropriate and potentially unsafe therapy. Prescribers should always be prepared to reconsider a diagnosis and be able critically to appraise the information on which any diagnosis is made.

Therapeutic decisions in primary care are frequently made on a heuristic basis (intelligent rules of thumb) (Essex, 1994). The 'rules' reflect the health beliefs and experience of that practitioner and the nature of a problem may be elucidated over several consultations. The contrast between the nature of the family practitioner and hospital decision-making is illustrated in Table 2.1. Although an over-simplification, it serves to illustrate the fundamentally different environment within which the primary care practitioner is required to operate. Inevitably, there will be many circumstances in

Table 2.1. The polar circumstances of the decision-making environment in general practice and hospital and their potential influence on the accuracy of diagnostic labels

Issue	General / Family Practice	Hospital
Problem type	Unselected	Selected
Who makes decisions	Alone, in isolation	Often made with other doctors and colleagues
Influence of knowledge of the family	Decisions affected	Decisions often made with no knowledge of the family
Time available	Short consultations, little time	More time to take history and fully examine
Seriousness and urgency of problem	Decision made by GP outside hospital	Decided on before admission or referral
Type of problem	Worried about something, Minor illness, Chronic disease	Mainly major illness, Chronic disease
Stage in natural history the disease is seen	Often early	Usually late
Type and range of decisions	Very broad, with several problems presented at once	More focused, often on an organ or system, depending on specialty
Review of decisions	Easily reviewed	Hard to review after discharge

which the hospital doctor will practise in a way that is similar to the family practitioner – and vice versa. The nature of this decision-making process, in which a definite diagnosis is not always made, has implications for the certainty with which diagnostic labels can be applied, and how much it can be depended on. For example, at what point should chest pain on exercise be labelled angina? The implication of using this diagnosis in primary care is that that patient may be coded into the practice computer system as having ischaemic heart disease. Consequently, they may be called in for all sorts of preventive procedures that may or may not be appropriate. To give a specific example: a patient in his 50s, a lifelong smoker, started getting chest pain walking up a steep cobbled street. He was advised not to smoke and given GTN tablets to take to relieve the pain. (GTN is glyceryl trinitrate, a vasodilator and standard treatment for angina.) It appeared to control the pain. Later, this person was started on aspirin, then later on he was started on a β-blocker (blood pressure drug, which also helps control angina); more recently his cholesterol was checked and found to be high and he was started on a statin. Some 25 years later he is alive and well and has had no deterioration at all in his symptoms. It is hard to tell if he has been treated successfully or really has angina at all.

In all circumstances we need to think critically about the diagnosis or we take risks with patient safety with no clear advantage to the patient.

Issuing a safe prescription

Many factors need to be taken into account before prescribing. A prescriber needs to include in their appraisal:

1. The age of the patient or sometimes the weight can be important in deciding the correct dose. This is particularly important in the very young and older people.

Whilst it is obvious that immature and ageing organ systems will behave differently, age-related prescribing safety problems are still common. It is essential always to check doses unless you are very familiar with doses in any age group. For example, in children, small doses of opiates can be fatal, and iron provides an example of something fairly innocuous in adults, but much more toxic in young children. Doses of tricyclic anti-depressants, which could cause minimal side effects in the young adult population, can cause drowsiness and increase the risk of falls in the elderly.

2.   Female gender:

   (a)   Are they taking the oral or other contraceptive?
   (b)   Are they pregnant or trying to conceive?
   (c)   Are they breast feeding?

Some therapies can interact with oral contraceptives and potentially result in an unwanted pregnancy. These include anti-epileptics and antibiotics.

Women who are trying to conceive, are pregnant or breast feeding need to avoid a wide range of medications. As far as possible, all non-essential medicines should be avoided at the time of conception and in early pregnancy. Other medications can be more important to avoid in the last trimester of pregnancy or prior to delivery. The British National Formulary (BNF) (British Medical Association, 2008) and other drug dictionaries contain special sections on pregnancy and breast feeding and it is well worth looking in these sections prior to prescribing.

3.   Ethnicity can affect the choice of medication in some diseases, and be associated with an increased risk of side effects

Ethnicity can also influence prescribing safety (see Chapter 5). For example, some Mediterranean races are more prone to a disease called thalassaemia. In the 'carrier' condition people can have microcytic anaemia (but not be iron deficient) and suffer from iron overload as a result of incorrect prescribing of iron. Some black people may respond differently to anti-hypertensive therapy, and some guidelines recommend different therapeutic options.

4.   Impairment or loss of function of certain body systems can affect prescribing safety. Of particular importance are:

   (a)   Reduction in kidney function
   (b)   Impaired liver metabolism

Changes in kidney and liver function can affect drugs excreted or metabolized by either of these organs. Such influences are common and are often clinically significant. Drug formularies such as the BNF list in separate appendices drugs where there may be potential hazards, or those which must be prescribed with caution in such circumstances. For example, the anticoagulant Warfarin can have its metabolism affected by other drugs which are metabolized in the liver.

5.   Other drugs which might interact with the proposed therapy

Drug interactions are also common. Prescribers need to be mindful of these and either expect to have to look them up (there is another appendix listing interactions in the BNF), or use prescribing software which lists them. These lists can never be exhaustive, but are a good starting point. However, they need interpretation in a particular context. For example, steroids cause salt and water retention and may not be the first choice of drug for treating someone who is already taking a diuretic. However, using steroids to treat an exacerbation of asthma they may be justified – the benefits of use vastly outweighing the risks. Or where a small amount of a topical steroid is being used short term, the interaction flag which appears can rightly be ignored.

6.   Other clinical diagnoses which can affect mediation choice

Co-morbidities can affect medication choice. For example, B-blockers used to treat hypertension and ischaemic heart disease may be contraindicated in asthma, where they may induce wheeze. Psychiatric co-morbidities can be much more complex to manage. Some schemes to support safe prescribing are in place. For example, patients who regularly take 'overdoses' may be prescribed short duration prescriptions issued weekly by a local pharmacy.

7.   Lifestyle

Lifestyle can influence the safety of medications. For example, alcohol can have enhanced sedative properties when taken with a range of anti-depressant and analgesic medications. Some drugs have increased risks of side effects among smokers: for example, dyspepsia may be more common in smokers on anti-inflammatory drugs.

8.   Cognitive function

Much of the developed world faces the challenge of how to care for its ageing population who carry an increasing burden of chronic disease. It can be extremely difficult to prescribe for elderly patients with impaired cognitive function; it is often uncertain to the prescriber whether this impaired function is temporary or permanent and sometimes the patient's assurances are a form of confabulation. Many elderly patients have several co-morbidities and are on multiple medications. The decision to prescribe should be based, in the first instance, on the prescriber's own observations and where appropriate these should be checked out by other members of the team. Aids to improving patient concordance may need to be considered, for example, improved labelling, appropriate containers or tray systems, which bring together all the medication needed to be taken at a particular time of day in a multi-compartment box or tray.

9.   Can the patient give consent for treatment?

Most patients give consent for their treatment. Where the patient cannot give consent, whatever is known about their wishes (if set out in advance of their illness or current condition) should be followed wherever possible, fitting in with the wishes of their relatives. If there is doubt, then clinicians should discuss this with their colleagues. Where doubt remains, or there is dispute, then if needed, legal advice should be sought. Most clinicians would initially do this through their professional body or medical defence society. Increasingly healthcare organisations seek the views of the courts as to whether continuing or discontinuing treatment is appropriate for a patient unable to give consent.

10.   Allergies and adverse reactions to drugs

Allergies and adverse reactions to medications are common. They need to be taken into account as part of the appraisal with regards to how safe it is to prescribe. These adverse reactions can vary from the minor and inconvenient to major and potentially life-threatening. Problems are not just restricted to new or expensive drugs, for example, the authors have looked after patients who have become severely anaemic in response to taking aspirin as prophylaxis in ischaemic heart disease.

Appropriate follow-up

Follow-up of patients is essential. Many of the unnecessary hospital admissions described above result from inadequate follow-up or monitoring. It is helpful if there is management continuity across a practice or clinic. For example, in our practice, we follow up all our stable hypertensive patients twice a year. Generally, they see the practice nursing team and the Primary care physician alternately.

On initiation of new treatment regimes, follow-up instructions should be part of a 'safety-net' put in place for all patients. It should reflect what is appropriate for that patient and their particular context. Dose adjustment of existing medication is also a time when a revised safety-net should be put in place. For example, a patient starting an angiotensin converting enzyme inhibitor (ACE-I) should be warned that the first dose may over-lower their blood pressure. People having their dosage of ACE-I adjusted should have their renal function checked as occasionally these medicines can have an adverse effect on kidney function.

Review and the 'safety-net' should things go wrong

Prescribers and their organizations should have a system which ensures a standard approach to supporting patients – we suggest adopting the approach suggested by Neighbour. In his classic book on the clinical consultation, he suggests there are five checkpoints that should be visited in each consultation (Neighbour, 2005). The one that is most relevant to prescribing safety is Checkpoint 4 'Safety-netting'. In a nutshell this is:

'Considering what may go wrong, or play out differently and planning accordingly.'

Prescribing errors and problems with drug safety are currently systemic problems within healthcare and we should tailor our advice for each consultation.

Knowing what to do if things go wrong

Prescribers need to be prepared to deal with problems that might arise when they prescribe. Prescribers who administer medication on their premises (e.g. give emergency drugs in their clinic or patients' homes or provide immunisations) need a higher level of preparedness than those who simply issue prescriptions that are dispensed elsewhere.

Prescribers should always be trained to manage emergencies and have access to appropriate medications and the other equipment needed to deal with adverse reactions.

Training should include the following:

1. Plan and rehearse according to circumstances

   (a) Take into account the distance of premises from other medical facilities.
   (b) The type of prescribing carried out (e.g. drug trials).
   (c) The physical layout of facilities (e.g. stairs when no lift, can a stretcher be moved along the corridor).
   (d) Providing ready access to medication to treat anaphylaxis and other drug-related emergencies.
   (e) The minimum number of people who must be on the premises. For example: a medium-sized general practice may say that there must be two people trained in resuscitation, and one other able to given an appropriate message to the ambulance service, phone ahead to the local accident and emergency department and ensure a clear route for the ambulance service if they need to attend.

2. Cardiopulmonary resuscitation and circulatory support

   (a) Basic life support (BLS) tested annually is the minimum standard.
   (b) Non-clinical staff should also be trained in BLS and how to support clinical staff involved in resuscitation.

3. How to summon help and team work

   (a) A telephone and regularly updated telephone numbers, including that of the local admitting hospital, should be available in all rooms.
   (b) Call other healthcare professionals and staff (e.g. panic buttons, call over the phone system).

4. Equipment to manage emergencies

   (a) Skills and appropriate equipment to maintain an airway.
   (b) Skills and appropriate equipment (e.g., ambu bag) to support breathing and to have oxygen available.
   (c) Equipment to establish venues access where needed and IV fluids.
   (d) Treatment for anaphylaxis and other common emergencies readily available on an emergency tray.
   (e) Where administering drugs at home appropriate drugs and equipment should be carried by the prescriber.

Access to up-to-date prescribing information

Many factors need to be taken into account before issuing a safe prescription. Prescribing safely therefore requires time and space for the careful consideration of these factors.

Miller (1956) back in the 1950s established that most people could only process seven items of information simultaneously: Miller's number. Exceptionally, people can handle two more items; however, some people can only handle five. 'The magical number seven plus or minus two (…) limits our capacity for processing information.' (Miller, 1956). The implication of Miller's hypothesis is that many complex prescribing decisions may exceed our usual capacity to process information. Consequently when prescribing in complex cases (e.g. an elderly person with several diagnoses and on multiple medications), we need time often directly with the patient; and with access to that person's medical records, including existing medications and access to prescribing data. The minimum data that should be available are the following:

1. Patient information

   (a) Their wishes, in respect to the proposed prescription.
   (b) History from the patient – face-to-face, by telephone and sometimes in writing.
   (c) The patient's medical record.

2. A drug dictionary

   (a) British National Formulary.
   (b) Children's British National Formula.
   (c) MIMS (Monthly Index of Medical Specialities).
   (d) Data sheet compendium.

3. Access to guidelines

   (a) Management of common long-term conditions.
   (b) Relevant specialist areas, e.g. end-of-life care.

Without access to these information sources and the time to process the information, prescribing is potentially dangerous. Use Miller's number to assess whether you are trying to process too great a volume of information. For example, you are late for your clinic, and also trying to remember you are due to phone another patient back. You are stopped in the corridor and asked to prescribe for a young male adult who has backache keeping him awake after a busy weekend gardening; he is not on any medications and has no history of indigestion. Here, you are being asked to process five items of information:

1. patient characteristics = young male;
2. reasonable grounds for therapy = backache keeping him awake;
3. patient's wishes = patient wants a prescription;
4. no alarm symptoms = a causation of backache which is reasonable;
5. no obvious contraindication = no medicines to interact and no dyspepsia (always worth checking before prescribing anti-inflammatories).

Many of our prescription requests are more complicated and many elderly people have multiple diagnosis and are already on many medications. The clinician should steadily work through the three steps outlined above (1. the patient; 2. relevant drug and prescribing information; and 3. guidelines for best practice). The problem needs to be broken down into constituent parts, none of which is likely to involve processing more than Miller's number of items of information.

Clinical governance and systems to ensure safe prescribing

There are two key themes in ensuring we are minimizing the risks, and prescribing as safely as possible. These are:

(1) Trying to ensure you are part of a safe system. This is the responsibility of every professional and can't be ignored just because of organizational or health system inertia. We recommend that prescribing safety is appraised using a

Donabedian approach looking at how structures, processes and outcomes support or provide evidence of safe prescribing.

(2)   Developing the characteristics of a lifelong learner. This may include the formal requirements to participate in review of critical incidents and clinical audit as part of appraisal or revalidation – but we would urge prescribers to work beyond this and constantly critically appraise their prescribing.

System issues in prescribing

To ensure that as a prescriber you are part of a safe system, we recommend that all prescribers evaluate the structures, process and outcome measures in place to ensure they are prescribing safely (Donabedian, 1966).

1.   **Structures.** The 'structures' are the physical things in place to promote prescribing safety. They include: physical aspects of the prescription such as a patient identifier and more recently the obligation to include the age of the patient; access to a drug formulary (we would recommend the BNF in the UK), guidelines and other relevant information at every point where prescribing might take place; physical systems that mean that the advice and help of colleagues can be obtained where needed and to deal with emergencies. Importantly, they must include systems which allow prescribing to be audited within its clinical context and allow outlying prescribing behaviour or clinical outcomes to be monitored. In the UK, legislation (successive Health and Social Care Acts) has placed the duty of 'Clinical Governance' on chief executives of health services and later on all healthcare providers. Additionally, other statutory bodies exist to define best practice (NICE – National Institute for Health and Clinical Excellence) and for inspection (the Care Quality Commission).

2.   **Processes.** Clinicians and health services need to have processes in place to ensure safe prescribing. For the clinician, this may include feedback on their consultation style to ensure that they include checking for contraindications and interactions. Where needed, training or mentorship should be provided. Health service managers need to ensure that processes are in place, which can be realistically carried out in the time available to the clinician. The duty of clinical governance means that patients should be treated according to best practice, as defined within the literature or within guidance issued by bodies such as NICE. There needs to be a culture of reviewing prescribing practice including prescribing errors. This should include taxonomy for reporting prescribing safety issues. Ideally, a single taxonomy should be adopted to allow comparisons between units and health systems. However, it may also need to reflect the needs of each specialty and the context within which it delivers healthcare. The Canadian primary care taxonomy for errors and adverse events is an exemplar (Jacobs *et al.*, 2007). Data should be in the public domain so that expert patients can make rational choices based on as much information as possible.

3.   **Outcome measures.** We all need to have our prescribing monitored for 'hard' outcomes (including death or unnecessary admissions). However, surrogate outcome measures (surrogate markers are those associated with poor outcome)

of prescribing safety may be measured more easily and potentially allow interventions to take place ahead of prescribing problems. An audit of practice or clinic records for known problems is a good way to start, and, again, should be seen as part of good professional practice rather than as any form of criticism. Evaluation of prescribing outcomes should generally be seen as a formative process. It should be led largely from within clinical teams; but should also be subject to external scrutiny. Prescribing advisors are well placed to carry out this work in a community setting, and ward pharmacists within secondary care. Audit-based education may provide an appropriate vehicle for combining the monitoring of process and outcome measures with learning (de Lusignan, 2002).

Lifelong learning

Prescribing is limited to clinical professionals. Clinical professionals have a duty to keep themselves updated as part of their requirements for registration by their professional body. The pace of change in pharmaceuticals and their guidelines for safe use are so great that it is essential to ensure appropriate support mechanisms are in place. For example, β-blockers once thought to be contraindicated in heart failure are now part of guidelines for best practice; anti-depressants once thought safe in adolescence are now known to be associated with an increased suicide risk. Individuals and organizations need to implement appropriate knowledge management strategies (de Lusignan, 2002).

We recommend that the following components should be in place.

1. **Appraisal/re-validation.** Prescribers should be part of a system of appraisal and revalidation. Whilst there is no evidence-base that links these activities to increased prescribing safety, we believe they create a mechanism for the formal review of issues relating to prescribing safety. The challenge for these processes is to make recommendations that tackle unsafe elements of current systems.

2. **Continuing professional development (CPD)/Personal development plan (PDP).** Your CPD/PDP should include an appraisal of the structures, processes and outcomes in place to ensure safe prescribing, and list the issues you plan to address in the coming year. Be realistic, you can't evaluate everything every year. However, list concerns which have arisen and discuss with your appraiser or mentor how to address them. Make sure you have the necessary training to take advantage of the safe systems in place to ensure prescribing safety.

3. **Mentorship/supervision by someone who is a current prescriber.** It is important that all prescribers have a mentor or supervisor that they can talk to about prescribing issues or the prescribing system they work within. Where the line manager is not a prescriber, an appropriate additional person should be identified.

4. **Team-working.** Team-working is dealt with as an issue in its own right in the next section. In summary, all prescribers should work in teams. These teams might be virtual or physical. For example, specialist asthma nurses might meet

physically very infrequently, but keep in regular email contact with regard to prescribing safety or other issues. Teams are essential for sharing experiences (for support) and socializing tacit understanding into explicit knowledge (the process whereby know-how gets shared and then included into usual practice). The culture of the team should be one of open sharing of prescribing practice including prescribing errors. There should be mechanisms in place for reviewing individual cases, for example, critical incidents reporting; as well as audit of care across populations including individuals prescribing practice. Practitioners should be able to critically appraise the quality of their team-working (Shaw *et al.*, 2005).

Communication and team-working

Communication and team-working are essential for safe prescribing. Communication is important within the local team (for mutual support and developing understanding); in the local medical records; in the shared record; and when reviewing safety issues (either at the individual patient or practice/system level).

Prescribers have to face pressure to prescribe unnecessarily or where there is a scant evidence base. For example, primary care physicians come under considerable pressure from their patients to prescribe 'slimming tablets' yet are mindful that these medicines have very poor success rates. Likewise, prescribers might have patients refuse to take a medicine that the prescriber felt was really of benefit to them. Although respecting patient autonomy is essential if a prescriber consults with someone who has had two previous heart attacks; has had a coronary revascularization and his current cholesterol is significantly raised. The person refuses lipid lowering therapy and this inevitably creates tensions. Prescribers need to work in teams with opportunities for informal discussion of problems and issues. Isolated practice should be avoided.

Keeping good medical records is essential for prescribing safety. We have discussed above how many factors can influence safe prescribing. A medical record needs to include data on all of these if we are to guarantee to avoid prescribing safety issues. Obviously, there can be some short cuts – the well person, who has had no operations or illnesses, not on any medicines or allergic to any – is a low-risk person for whom to prescribe. However, many people have complex medical problems – and we need to construct safe records to work from or we risk perpetuating a system that continues to have the high rate of errors reported at the start of this chapter.

Increasingly, clinical records are shared. Historically different professions and institutions kept separate records, only sharing information where needed. Now shared records are more common either on paper (e.g., records kept at home during end-of-life care), or electronic where all information is shared across a single linked computerized medical record. We need to learn how to work with shared and patient-held records – online records accessed and edited by the patient are likely to become increasingly widespread.

A safe prescriber will critically appraise the medical record and *not* take its contents as sacrosanct. Much of what is important in team-working has been set out in the sections above; however, the importance of working with pharmacists has not been sufficiently stressed. Pharmacists contribute to safer prescribing in two ways: (1) Scrutiny of individual prescriptions; (2) Feedback on prescribing practice. Sometimes, these two roles are combined; this is often the case in hospital practice. However, in the community they are often separate. The community pharmacist scrutinizes the prescriptions prior to dispensing them, and the local health service prescribing advisors look at prescribing practice. Over our years as prescribers, we estimate that the local community pharmacist will need to discuss two to four prescriptions per week with Primary care prescribers or other members of the practice team. Many of the enquiries are about non-safety issues such as duration, preparation availability, etc. However, around 20% are about safety issues. Often, these are risk–benefit issues already taken into account by the prescriber – but in an important minority these are genuine safety issues which would otherwise be missed.

Decision support and using technology to support safer prescribing

Electronic prescribing offers four potential benefits: completeness and legibility of prescriptions; the option of linkage to prescribing data; decision support and electronic transmission to the pharmacy to speed up the dispensing process.

1. **Computer-generated prescriptions.** Computer-generated prescriptions are nearly always legible and have more complete information. An electronic prescription won't print without full patient information, dosage, etc. The problems with written prescriptions are well known (Gommans, 2008) and computerization removes many of these.

2. **Linking to prescribing data – improved 'information retrieval'.** Computerized prescriptions can link to information (e.g. electronic BNF) and allow rapid 'information retrieval' (IR). Clinicians commonly use a paper drug dictionary to look up information; some of our computerized colleagues continue to do this as they can then look things up on paper, while the whole drug list is displayed in front of them on their computer.

3. **Computerized decision support systems (CDSS).** Computerized decision support systems (CDSS) are described as basic or advanced. Basic CDSS include the flagging of drug allergy and duplicate medications. Advanced CDSS should link medication with disease, and identify much more advanced forms of therapeutic duplication – for example, within drug groups. Hitherto, many alerts designed to improve prescribing safety have been of low clinical significance and have been ignored; whilst alerts are in theory a great thing, most are overridden (Lasser *et al.*, 2006; Shah, 2006). CDSS have also been implemented to support lower-cost prescribing choices, but are sometimes a distraction rather than a positive aid to prescribing safety (de Lusignan, 2008). There are exceptions; for example, the use of computerized alerts has been shown to improve prescribing in the elderly. The key appears to be high degrees of selectivity of alerts and constant improvement.

Despite its obvious advantages, the implementation of computerized prescribing has been variable. Repeat prescribing took off in UK general practice because it was one of the few computer functions that saved Primary care physicians' time.

Computerized physician order entry (CPOE) has had a much more variable rate of adoption internationally. Although potentially offering scope to reduce prescribing errors, implementing technological systems into complex organizations is problematic. Some technologies, such as bar coding, help reduce patient identification errors, but like other technological innovations add to prescribing administration time.

Summary

The approach that we recommend to achieve safe prescribing is similar to that advocated by the World Health Organization and extended by Pollock *et al.* (2007). We have stressed that prescribers must be sensitive to a large number of factors and these will often exceed Miller's number. Where a clinician is likely to be asked to integrate more than seven items to form a rational decision, we recommend they take interruption-free time and break the decision down into manageable components.

However, in addition to promoting safe prescribing at the point of care, we feel that developing safe systems is probably of greater importance in the long term – given the high levels of prescribing safety issues. This is particularly important in societies where there is an ever-increasing disease burden in an ageing population. System problems can be addressed at the local clinic or team level as well as at the national or health system level. They are everyone's responsibility.

Technology has an important role in improving prescribing safety and changing the nature of the prescribing task; but it is no panacea. Prescribers will increasingly know how to use these tools rather than be the holders of information. Patients will have equal access to these information sources. Clinicians will work in partnership with their patients to help guide them to the appropriate weighting to give different sources of information.

Advances in pharmaceuticals have made an enormous contribution to improved health over the last 50 years. It could be argued that this contribution has been greater than any other branch of medicine. However, in our enthusiasm to adopt new products that do more for our patients, the establishment of processes to ensure they are used as safely as possible has not kept pace.

References

Aylin P, Best N, Bottle A, Marshall C. (2003). Following Shipman: a pilot system for monitoring mortality rates in primary care. *Lancet*, **362**(9382), 485–91.

British Medical Association (2008). Royal Pharmaceutical Society of Great Britain. British National Formulary (BNF) 56. *RPS London*, URL: http://www.bnf.org.

Bates DW. (2005). The Critical Care Safety Study: The incidence and nature of adverse events and serious medical errors in intensive care. *Crit Care Med*, **33**(8), 1694–700.

Bates DW, Gandhi TK. (2006). Improving acceptance of computerized prescribing alerts in ambulatory care. *Journal of the American Medical Information Association*, **13**(1), 5–11.

Borgheini G. (2003). The bioequivalence and therapeutic efficacy of generic versus brand-name psychoactive drugs. *Clinical Therapy*, **25**(6), 1578–92.

Committee on Quality of Health Care in America. (2000). *To Err is Human: Building a Safer Health System*.

Washington, DC: National Academy Press. URL: http://books.nap.edu/catalog/9728.html.

Committee on Quality of Health Care in America, (2001). *Institute of Medicine/ Crossing the Quality Chasm: A New Health System for the 21st Century.* Washington, DC: National Academy Press, URL: http://www.nap.edu/catalog.php?record_id=10027.

de Lusignan S. (2007). An educational intervention, involving feedback of routinely collected computer data, to improve cardiovascular disease management in UK primary care. *Methods in Information Medicine*, **46**(1), 57–62.

de Lusignan S. (2008). Prescribing support software recommends more expensive prescriptions. *Information Primary Care*, **16**(1), 61–2.

de Lusignan S, Pritchard K, Chan T. (2002). A knowledge-management model for clinical practice. *Journal of Postgraduate Medicine*, **48**(4), 297–303.

de Lusignan S. (2003). The National Health Service and the internet. *Journal of the Royal Society of Medicine*, **96**(10), 490–3.

Donabedian A. (1966). Evaluating the quality of medical care. *Milbank Memorial Fund Quarterly*, **44**(3), Suppl, 166–206.

Essex B. (1994). *Doctor's Dilemmas and Decisions*. London: BMJ Books.

Fullerton SE. (1984). Parallel imports: a pharmacist's viewpoint. *British Medical Journal, (Clinical Research Education)*, **288**(6433), 1778–9.

Food and Drugs Administration (FDA). Electronic Orange Book: Approved drug products with therapeutic equivalence calculations. URL: http://www.fda.gov/cder/ob/

Franklin BD, O'Grady K, Donyai P, Jacklin A, Barber N. (2007). The impact of a closed-loop electronic prescribing and administration system on prescribing errors, administration errors and staff time: a before-and-after study. *Quality Safety in Health Care*, **16**(4), 279–84.

Gommans J, McIntosh P, Bee S, Allan W. (2008). Improving the quality of written prescriptions in a general hospital: the influence of 10 years of serial audits and targeted interventions. *International Medical Journal*, **38**(4), 243–8.

International Pharmacy Federation (FIP). Good pharmacy practice (GPP) in developing countries. *Recommendations for stepwise implementation*. URL: http://www.fip.nl/www2/pdf/gpp/GPP_CPS_Report.pdf

Jacobs S, O'Beirne M, Derflingher LP, Vlach L, Rosser W, Drummond N. (2007). Errors and adverse events in family medicine: developing and validating a Canadian taxonomy of errors. *Canadian Family Physician*, **53**(2), 271–6.

Koppel R, Leonard CE, Localio AR, Cohen A, Auten R, Strom BL. (2008). Identifying and quantifying medication errors: evaluation of rapidly discontinued medication orders submitted to a computerized physician order entry system. *Journal of the American Medical Information Association*, **15**(4), 461–5.

Kunac DL, Reith DM. (2005). Identification of priorities for medication safety in neonatal intensive care. *Drug Safety*, **28**(3), 251–61.

Lasser KE, Allen PD, Woolhandler SJ, Himmelstein DU, Wolfe SM, Bor DH. (2002). Timing of new black box warnings and withdrawals for prescription medications. *Journal of the American Medical Association*, **287**(17), 2215–20.

Lasser KE, Seger DL, Yu DT *et al.* (2006). Adherence to black box warnings for prescription medications in outpatients. *Archives of Internal Medicine*, **166**(3), 338–44.

Neighbour R. (2005). *The Inner Consultation*, 2nd Edition. Oxford: Radcliffe.

Miller G. (1956). The magical number seven, plus or minus two: some limits on our capacity for processing information. *The Psychological Review*, **63**, 81–97.

Mott DA, Cline RR. (2002). Exploring generic drug use behavior: the role of prescribers and pharmacists in the opportunity for generic drug use and generic substitution. *Medical Care*, **40**(8), 662–74.

NICE (2008). Respiratory tract infections – antibiotic prescribing; Prescribing of antibiotics for self-limiting respiratory tract infections in adults and children in primary care. *NICE Clinical Guideline 69*. London: NICE.

NPSA (2007). *Safety in doses: medication safety incident in the NHS: The fourth report from the Patient Safety Observatory*. London: NPSA.

Nuckols TK, Bell DS, Liu H, Paddock SM, Hilborne LH. (2007). Rates and types of events reported to established incident reporting systems in two US hospitals. *Quality Safety Health Care*, **16**(3), 164–8.

Pallás CR, De-la-Cruz J, Del-Moral MT, Lora D, Malalana MA. (2008). Improving the quality of medical prescriptions in neonatal units. *Neonatology*, **93**(4), 251–6.

Rosser W, Dovey S, Bordman R, White D, Crighton E, Drummond N. (2005). Medical errors in primary care: results of an international study of family practice. *Can Fam Physician*, **51**, 386–7.

Shaw A, de Lusignan S, Rowlands G. (2005). Do primary care professionals work as a team: a qualitative study. *Journal of Interprofessional Care*, **19**(4), 396–405.

Smith DH, Perrin N, Feldstein A *et al.* (2006). The impact of prescribing safety alerts for elderly persons in an electronic medical record: an interrupted time series evaluation. *Archives Internal Medicine*, **166**(10), 1098–104.

Solomon DH, Schneeweiss S, Glynn RJ *et al.* (2004). Relationship between selective cyclooxygenase-2 inhibitors and acute myocardial infarction in older adults. *Circulation*, **109**(17), 2068–73.

Panoskaltsis N. (2006). Cytokine storm in a phase 1 trial of the anti-CD28 monoclonal antibody TGN1412. *New England Journal of Medicine*, **355**(10), 1018–28.

Thomsen LA, Winterstein AG, Søndergaard B, Haugbølle LS, Melander A. (2007). Systematic review of the incidence and characteristics of preventable adverse drug events in ambulatory care. *Annals of Pharmacotherapy*, **41**(9), 1411–26.

World Health Organization, URL: (http://www.who.int/medicines/publications/essentialmedicines/en/

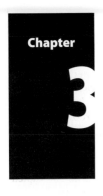

Chapter 3

Safety in dispensing

Imogen Savage

When someone is prescribed a medicine, he or she expects the doctor to have made the right choice, and to receive what the doctor has ordered. Ensuring that these expectations are fulfilled is a fundamental part of the pharmacist's job, but most people waiting for prescriptions are probably unaware of the routines that are designed to keep them safe. Instead, they may watch staff at work and wonder why dispensing a few tablets can take so long. As for prescribing (Nemeth & Cook, 2005), the routine technical work that dispensary staff do is hiding in plain sight. It only becomes visible when something goes wrong and a mistake is made.

Pharmacists have a professional responsibility to ensure the well-being and safety of their patients and the public (RPSGB, 2007). As part of this, they should assess every prescription presented for dispensing to determine its suitability for the patient, and should also make sure that the patient is given the information and advice needed to enable the safe and effective use of the medicine that has been ordered.

This chapter will do the following:

- Explain the steps in the basic prescription management process that take place in any UK dispensary. The issue of the dispensed medicines and the provision of information and advice will not be considered.
- Consider key research evidence for the effectiveness of this process.
- Discuss the possible impact of new information and communication technologies.
- Consider implications for the education and training of future pharmacists.

Scope and terminology

This chapter will consider current UK community and hospital pharmacy practice. It will use the term 'doctor' but recognizes that other healthcare workers (including some pharmacists) can now prescribe.

Dispensing mistakes that are detected after the medicine leaves the dispensary will be called dispensing errors. Mistakes that are picked up during the checking process within the dispensary will be referred to as 'near misses'.

The screening routine described in the next section is intended to check three aspects of safety: (1) the legality and authority of the medication order, (2) the prescribing, and (3) the physical assembly of the medicine that has been ordered. Pharmacists often refer to (2) as 'the clinical check' and (3) as the 'technical check' or the 'final check'.

Care sectors and prescription types

Prescriptions are written in two main settings: primary and secondary care. In both sectors, the bulk of prescribing and dispensing is done under the National Health Service,

Medication Safety: An Essential Guide, ed. Molly Courtenay and Matt Griffiths. Published by Cambridge University Press. © M. Courtenay and M. Griffiths 2009.

and the majority of prescriptions will be computer generated (i.e. typed). However, prescriptions are also written in private hospitals, in private medical and dental practice, and in a growing range of non-NHS clinics. Primary care physicians (GPs) may also write private prescriptions as some medicines are not available under the NHS.

In hospitals, the majority of prescriptions will be handwritten. The design of inpatient drug charts and outpatient prescriptions will vary between Trusts and between private hospital groups.

In primary care, NHS prescribing is done on the standard FP10 prescription form, and the majority of prescriptions will be computer printed with handwritten scripts only produced away from the surgery, for example, on urgent house calls. Most private (non-NHS) prescribing is in handwriting on the prescriber's practice-headed notepaper.

The bulk of prescriptions which are not written in hospital are dispensed in Britain's hospital pharmacies. These can be divided into two main groups: independent businesses and pharmacies that are part of a chain or large corporation.

Most hospital Trusts have their own pharmacy department that will deal with all inpatient and discharge medicine needs. Depending on staffing, hospital pharmacies may also dispense prescriptions from outpatient clinics. Alternatively, patients can be given an FP10 to take to their local community pharmacy.

Hospital pharmacists will therefore normally only handle prescriptions from their own NHS Trust or private hospital group. Community pharmacies will be presented with a wider range of prescription formats.

The basic prescription management process

When a prescription is presented for dispensing, pharmacists and their staff will have a set routine – or standard operating procedure – to follow. This should be set out in writing so that all staff, including locums, know what is normal practice. The details of who does what may vary depending on the practice setting, but it is a fundamental rule that the pharmacist must see the prescription at some stage.

Receipt and validity check

In primary care, the initial receipt of a prescription is usually done by a medicines counter assistant, as it is at this point that any prescription charges will be collected. In hospital pharmacies dispensing outpatient prescriptions, this may be done by a clerk.

The prescription is then passed to a pharmacist or dispensing technician, who will first check that the prescription is signed by someone who is authorized to prescribe the medicines, and that it is in date. Unsigned or undated orders are not legally valid. Shah et al. (2001) found a small proportion of GP prescriptions presented to three community pharmacies over 2 months were not dated, or not signed. The same can happen in hospital practice (Stubbs et al., 2004).

Most prescribers will be well known to staff; if there are any doubts, their status can be checked, for example, on the GMC website. There is little published data on the frequency of presentation of forged prescriptions but Primary Care Trusts have an early warning system for alerting pharmacies when a doctor's NHS prescription pad is stolen.

In hospital, it would be unusual to have a medication order which had not been written within 24 hours of presentation. In community practice, prescriptions must be dated within the last 6 months or 28 days for controlled drugs, to be legally valid orders. This validity check will protect a patient from using a medicine which may no longer be appropriate for them, but the prime purpose is to protect the public against fraud and illegal use of drugs, particularly those controlled under the Misuse of Drugs Act (CDs).

The extra legal requirements for the way that prescriptions for CD medicines such as strong opiates are written can cause inter-professional tension when prescriptions have to be returned for rewriting for technical reasons, even though the prescriber's intentions may be perfectly clear. In Shah *et al.*'s survey, 31 of the prescriptions presented did not comply with CD prescription-writing requirements.

The Shipman case led to redesign of pharmacy CD ledgers, so that receipts and supplies of each strength and form of a particular drug are now made on the same page. This should, hopefully, make unusual patterns of prescribing by individual doctors more obvious. The pharmacist who dispensed many of Dr Shipman's prescriptions was criticized by the chairman of the Shipman Inquiry for not questioning the 'extremely unusual' single doses of 30 mg diamorphine injection on 14 prescriptions for 13 patients. None of the patients had cancer and some were already dead.

Dr Shipman also often collected his prescriptions himself, which is unusual for a busy Primary care physician. Pharmacists dispensing CDs must now record the name of the person collecting the prescription, plus their own registration number.

Clinical check

As stated in the Introduction, pharmacists are required to assess every prescription before it is dispensed.

In community pharmacies, this clinical screen or check will usually be done in the dispensary as part of the dispensing process. In hospital pharmacies, the clinical check of an inpatient drug chart is usually done on the ward, and the order then transcribed for dispensing in the pharmacy. The clinical and dispensing checks therefore may take place some time apart and in different settings.

In hospitals, pharmacists check that inpatient medication orders for patients on their designated wards are legal, clear and clinically appropriate. They also check pre-admission drug histories, resolve problems and initiate supply of non-stock and discharge medicines.

Hospital pharmacists have more scope to amend or change prescriptions than do community pharmacists. Depending on local Trust policy, they may add or clarify information on drug names, doses and administration methods. They therefore have a wider safety remit than community pharmacists do, and may spend little or no time in the dispensary. Dean Franklin *et al.* (2007) have reported that pharmacists servicing one surgical ward in a teaching hospital spent over a third of their total work time on prescription screening activities, plus around 13% giving advice and information to staff and patients.

However, both hospital and community pharmacists have two basic professional duties: to check that the dose ordered is suitable for the patient's age and clinical condition, and to check that the medication ordered does not interfere with any other medication the patient is taking (Chapter 5). If they have any doubts, they should check with the prescriber. Pharmacists call this 'making an intervention'. Since 2005, pharmacists who are accredited to provide advanced services under the new pharmacy contract for England and Wales have been able to claim a fee for interventions that trigger a medication use review (Bellingham, 2004).

In hospitals, they may intervene if the drug chosen does not fit local or national protocols. In community practice, pharmacists will be familiar with the drugs and dose regimes that their local doctors use, but are less likely to query clinical choice unless prompted to do so by their PCT.

As part of the basic safety screen, pharmacists should also check that there are no obvious contraindications to the use of the drug (e.g. penicillin allergy; non-steroidal anti-inflammatory drug use in person with history of ulcers). This is much easier to do if there is access to the patient's medical notes. Community pharmacies do not yet have this access and must rely on their own knowledge of the patient, plus limited information recorded in the pharmacy medication records (PMRs).

Pharmacists first started to keep records of medication supplied to their regular prescription customers in the 1970s (Shulman et al., 1981). The development of dispensary computer technology facilitated wider adoption within the pharmacy profession, and now all pharmacies will maintain PMRs for all or most of their patients. At the time of writing (early 2008), these records are primarily a list of the patients' current and previous prescription medication, plus known allergies and contraindications. They will not provide a complete picture of what the patient is currently taking unless the patient always uses the same pharmacy, or always uses pharmacies in a chain such as Boots, which offers centralized electronic records.

Commercial dispensary software now routinely screens for drug–drug interactions. As with Primary care physicians' systems, there is variation in the quality of the decision support provided, with some systems warning for all interactions in the database, no matter what the level of clinical risk. Balon built his own system and used the British National Formulary classification to monitor interactions in his own pharmacy (Stevens & Balon, 1997). One in every 180 prescriptions presented for dispensing contained a potentially hazardous drug–drug interaction. Interestingly, few were changed after discussion with the prescriber because the patients were not actually experiencing clinical problems.

Dispensing accuracy check

The purpose of the dispensing check is to make sure that what has been supplied matches what has been ordered on the prescription. The paper prescription is set out on the bench, and each dispensed item is taken up in turn and compared against the written or printed order.

There are two main points at which mistakes happen during the physical dispensing process: when the medicine (product) is picked from the shelf and when the dispensing label is produced.

Dispensing labels are required by law in the UK. As well as showing what the medicine is, who it is for, and when and where it was dispensed, the label must also contain the instructions that the prescriber requests on how the medicine is to be taken or used. These printed instructions provide a memory aid for patients, who may not remember (or may not have been told) how much to take how often and for how long.

Label generation and product picking are often done by different people. In community pharmacies (Savage, 1999) it is often the pharmacist who calls up records, checks the prescription and generates labels, while a technician picks the medicines needed to fill the order, then affixes the labels to the final packs. In hospitals, where most prescriptions will be screened by a pharmacist before they reach the dispensary, an assistant technical officer (ATO) may pick stock and generate labels, with checking by a qualified pharmacy technician (Fitzpatrick *et al.,* 2005).

In most dispensaries there is a separate area or 'checking bench' where the assembled prescriptions are then set out in baskets to await a final accuracy check. The person doing the final check will be dictated by the SOP for that pharmacy; it may be an accredited checking technician, or it may be a pharmacist. Hospital dispensaries may be managed by technicians, who supervise dispensing by assistant technical officers (ATOs), but this is rare in community pharmacy. In larger dispensaries, one member of staff may be a designated 'final checker' and do only this throughout their shift.

It is accepted good practice that all dispensed medicines should be checked by an appropriately qualified second person before issue. The dispenser and the checker may both initial the dispensing label to show that this has been done. However, there will often be occasions when there is no second person to call on, for example, when working out-of-normal hours, and in smaller community pharmacies, which may have no dispensary help at all.

Dispensing check routines

The dispensing accuracy check is very much a 'taken for granted' process, and studies of dispensing errors rarely describe the normal routines used in the dispensaries.

There are two main schools of thought about how to check: start by checking the dispensing label against the prescription; and start by checking the product (medicine). The latter method saves time as, if the product is wrong, there is no point going any further because the prescription has to be redone and then rechecked.

Savage *et al.* (2007) have studied the final check process in 18 pharmacists, trained at ten UK schools of pharmacy and qualified from 1 to over 40 years. All had recent dispensary experience in the community and/or hospitals.

While product-first routines were more common than label-first routines, the order in which individual steps in the check were performed was highly individualized, with some pharmacists taking a more patient-focused approach than others. Most pharmacists worked down the list of medicines on the script. However, one subject deliberately did the reverse so he ended up 'back at the patient's name'.

Each pharmacist had his or her preparatory ritual, reading patient and/or prescriber information, counting the number of items, and setting packs in order, either in the basket or on the bench. For some, this initial scoping was a whole process check, with some clinical elements. One called this *'getting a feel'* for the prescription. They did this even though the prescription had already been screened for clinical problems by someone else.

Many checked with a pen in their hand. This could be used as a pointer to the label or script, or as a ruler, to underline a medicine order on the script. The product pack was also used by some in this way. Fingers and thumbs (held at each end of the label) were used to focus on elements of the label, usually the directions. Most said it was their normal practice to 'talk to themselves' while checking, especially if it was busy, or if they were tired.

Prescription screening: evidence for effectiveness

Worldwide there have been many studies describing the hospital and community pharmacists' role in checking for prescribing errors and adverse drug events.

In the UK, the routine screening of prescriptions has been part of ward pharmacy services since the late 1960s. This makes it difficult to test the effectiveness of the 'clinical check' in a controlled trial, as any wards not receiving a pharmacy service will be very different from wards that do.

However, data are available on the nature and frequency of the prescribing problems that pharmacists detect, both in hospital (Batty and Barber, 1992; Hawkey *et al.*, 1990; Stubbs *et al.*, 2004) and the community (Greene, 1995; Shah, 2001; Warner & Gerrett, 2005). The data for all of these studies were collected by pharmacists as part of their normal work, and all incidents would have required some intervention with the prescriber.

Table 3.1 summarizes the problems detected during routine screening. (Hospital-only interventions concerning drug level monitoring and adverse drug reactions have been omitted.) The percentages are approximations, as authors did not all use the same terms to classify incidents. Nevertheless, queries relating to dosing (product strength, number of dose units, dosing frequency) and the product (the drug and its pharmaceutical form) appear relatively consistent across the years. These types of error are also most frequently reported to the National Reporting and Learning System, forming over a quarter of all incidents reported (NPSA, 2007).

The comparison also suggests a reduction in drug and dose-related problems in more recent studies, although differences between hospital specialties need to be kept in mind. Figures for interventions concerning drug–drug interactions also suggest a decline. Some of this could reflect increased computerization, with better, more accessible, medication records. The emergence of new types of error, linked to increased use of computer records, can also be seen.

Greene's (1995) audit of prescription anomalies was done in 1987, at a time when dispensary computers, if used at all, were little more than labelling machines. Approximately 13% of pharmacists' queries concerned possible drug–drug interactions. Greene noted that, at that time, pharmacists queried interactions 'too often' and were not confident to take an independent decision on clinical significance.

More recent surveys (Shah *et al.*, 2001; Stubbs *et al.*, 2004; Warner & Gerrett, 2005) have reported a much lower proportion of drug–drug interactions. This probably reflects better decision support at both the GP and pharmacy level, plus, possibly, the impact of continuing professional education.

Shah and colleagues (2001) found significant variation between Primary care physicians and a higher incidence of errors on handwritten scripts. Chen *et al.* (2005) have carried out similar work, reporting 196 prescribing problems for 32 403 items dispensed. Incomplete or incorrect information on prescriptions accounted for two-thirds of problems.

Table 3.1. Prescription problems detected during routine screening (estimated from published data as % of total reports)

	Hospital			Community		
Authors	Batty & Barber	Hawkey *et al.*	Stubbs *et al.*	Greene	Shah *et al.*	Warner & Gerrett
Data collected (approx)	1990	1990	2003	1987	2001	2005
Setting	31 acute hospitals	6 acute / mental health	1 mental health	23 pharmacies	3 pharmacies	17 pharmacies
Time span	1 week	1 month	1 month	4 months	2 months	12 months
Total interventions reported	3758	769	211	214	2816	968
Drug and form	28%	22%	10%	24%	1%	6%
Dose/strength/ frequency	29%	37%	11%		10%	9%
Interactions/ contraindications	5%	13%	1.4%	13%		1%
Directions unclear			44%	30%	38%	5%
Illegal / illegible/ incomplete	9%	17%	15%		5%	
Prescribing not authorised	7%		12%		0.1%	
Duplication of medicines					0.6%	
Wrong patient					0.2%	2%

Differences in classification between authors make it difficult to separate out errors concerning the prescribed dose (a content error) from errors in instructions for administration (a labelling error). However, unclear or absent directions seem to remain a problem.

Errors and harm

Hawkey *et al.* (1990) questioned whether the hospital ward pharmacy services were cost-effective, pointing out that the effectiveness of the prescription screening process could not be assessed without information on how many errors the pharmacists missed. This is almost impossible to measure in a natural setting, although reports of actual, or potential, harm caused by errors that were not detected during routine screening can provide a proxy measure.

Many papers present the serious errors that pharmacists detect. In Hawkey's study, 4% of all prescribing interventions concerned dose-related errors which the authors judged could have led to significant harm. Stubbs *et al.* rated 11% of interventions on dosing or interactions as clinically significant. In primary care, Shah described 20 prescriptions with potentially hazardous directions, including one for methotrexate, plus

Wrong dose (1982)
Doctor prescribes Migril (contains ergotamine) as a regular treatment, when it should be used only for acute attacks of migraine, with a maximum of six tablets per week. Outcome: Patient takes medicine regularly every day as instructed and develops gangrene in both feet, requiring extensive surgery. Damages awarded against pharmacist (45%) and doctor (55%).

Wrong drug (1988)
Pharmacist misreads a handwritten prescription for an antibiotic (Amoxil) and dispenses an oral hypoglycaemic (Daonil) instead. Outcome: The patient, who was not diabetic, suffered irreversible brain damage. Damages awarded against prescriber (25%) and pharmacist/pharmacy company (75%).

Wrong strength (1998)
Baby prescribed peppermint water (Alder Hey formula) to treat colic. A pre-registration pharmacist uses too much concentrated chloroform water when making the preparation. The pharmacist signs the dispensing check slip without checking the actual dispensing. Outcome: When the medicine is given, the baby suffers a cardiac arrest, and subsequently dies. Pharmacist and trainee are cleared of manslaughter but fined for dispensing a defective medicine.

Figure 3.1. Prescription checking: Three cases where the process failed.

14 clinically significant drug interactions; a total of approximately 1% of all interventions made.

The vast majority of reports involving community pharmacy relate to dispensing, although harm resulting from failure to check drugs and doses has also occurred (see examples in Fig. 3.1).

Official reports do not consider the failure of prescription screening as a contributing factor to prescribing errors (NPSA, 2007). In the hospital setting, pharmacy chart review is only mentioned in relation to omitted medicines, resulting from delays in the supply to wards.

However, wrong dose, strength or frequency errors form over a third (38%) of the 92 cases of serious harm or death reported to the National Reporting and Learning Scheme between January 2005 and June 2006. Misunderstandings resulting from unclear, ambiguous or illegible medication orders are cited as common contributing factors. This suggests that, in these cases, the pharmacist's clinical check was either not done, or the errors were missed.

The incident most likely to cause harm was a patient receiving a drug to which s/he was allergic. Tuthill *et al.* (2004) reported that the patient's allergy status was not recorded on a quarter of inpatient drug charts audited at one London teaching hospital. Checking allergy documentation is part of the hospital pharmacist's role, but they may expect the prescriber to make the actual record.

Prescription assembly: evidence for the final dispensing check

Collecting evidence on the effectiveness of the dispensing check is more feasible than for the clinical screening process because mistakes that are not picked up internally within the dispensary are usually noticed by nurses (on wards) and by patients (in pharmacies or their own homes), and then reported. (However, the proportion that is missed entirely is unknown.)

The majority of published UK research uses self-reporting by pharmacy staff, either as part of an audit (Lynskey *et al.*, 2007; Ashcroft *et al.*, 2005; Beso *et al.*, 2005; Warner & Gerrett, 2005; Edmondson *et al.*, 2003) or via a centralized anonymous reporting system (Spencer & Smith, 1993; Roberts *et al.*, 2002). Only one study (Dean Franklin & O'Grady, 2007) has used observational methods to collect data.

Not all of these papers distinguish between errors which were picked up at the point of handing the medicine to a patient (still inside the pharmacy) and those only detected on the ward or in the patient's home. They do not all have the total number of items dispensed, and there are also differences in the way that errors are classified and grouped.

Table 3.2 summarizes findings from those research studies that allow the separation of content and labelling errors and near misses. Table 3.3 shows the proportions of errors detected (near misses) and missed by the final dispensing check.

Beso's hospital study suggests that around 1 in every 130 (0.02%:2.7%) dispensing errors is not picked up by the final dispensing check. Ashcroft and Edmondson's near miss figures reported are both very low in comparison to Dean Franklin's observed and probably reflect under-reporting.

In general, studies report more content errors than labelling errors. Comparing data from self-reports with the single observation study suggests a bias towards the reporting of wrong product errors, perhaps because these are perceived as more serious than labelling mistakes.

Errors and harm

Roberts *et al.* (2002) analysed 4380 dispensing error reports with outcome data from 89 hospital pharmacies between 1991 and 2001. Seven per cent of incidents were judged to have had a serious detrimental effect and there was one fatality. However, in the majority of medication errors that reach the patient, harm happens at the administration stage (NPSA, 2007). Of the 92 incidents resulting in severe harm or death reported between Jan 05 and June 06, only four could be attributed directly to the preparation or dispensing of the medicine concerned.

Table 3.2. Types of dispensing error detected and missed by the dispensing check (Summary of published data, as % of all errors made)

	Detected by final dispensing check		Not detected by dispensing check
	Self-report[a]	Observation[b]	Self-report[a]
Wrong content	41–58%	18%	19–66%
Wrong instructions	9–32%	28%	5–17%
Wrong patient	5–17%	11%	2–18%

[a]Spencer & Smith, 1993; Edmondson *et al.*, 2003; Ashcroft *et al.*, 2005; Beso *et al.*, 2005; Lynskey *et al.*, 2007.
[b]Dean Franklin & O'Grady, 2007.

Table 3.3. Proportions of errors detected and missed by the final dispensing check

Errors detected	Spencer et al. (1993)	Beso et al. (2005)	Edmondson et al. (2003)	Ashcroft et al. (2005)	Dean Franklin & O'Grady (2007)
Setting	Hospital	Hospital	Community	Community	Community
Timescale	6 months	2 weeks	8 weeks	4 weeks	2 days per site
N dispensaries	19	1	4	35	11
Content errors	42.4%	53.8%	58%	61%	51.6%
Labelling errors	57.6%	46.2%	23%	94 (33.5%)	46 (48.4%)
Total errors	1500	130	247	280	95
Total items dispensed	no data	4849	51 357	125 395	2859
Near miss rate		**2.7%**	**0.48%**	**0.22%**	**3.3%**
Errors missed					
Timescale	6 months	1 year	8 weeks	4 weeks	no data
Content errors	54%	66%	64%	56%	
Labelling errors	46%	34%	15%	30%	
Total errors	178	32	39	50	
Total items dispensed	1 002 095	194 584	51 357	125 395	
Error rate	**0.02%**	**0.02%**	**0.08%**	**0.04%**	

Percentages may not sum to 100 as some studies had additional error categories.

Dean Franklin *et al.* classified community pharmacy dispensing errors on their clinical significance. The majority of wrong content errors were judged to have 'moderate' clinical significance by a panel; labelling errors showed a greater range of potential severity with many being minor but at least one having the potential to cause real harm.

Perceived causes of errors

Table 3.4 shows the perceived causes of dispensing errors as reported in hospital (Spencer & Smith, 1993; Roberts *et al.*, 2001; Beso *et al.*, 2007) and community pharmacies (Lynskey *et al.*, 2007; Ashcroft *et al.*, 2005).

Picking errors linked to 'look-alike–sound-alike' product names and similar packs have been mentioned by all authors. In the hospital survey by Roberts *et al.* (2002), the ten drugs most commonly involved in dispensing errors accounted for 27% of serious or fatal outcomes. Most were because the wrong strength of the right drug had been picked. The DoH has issued guidelines on the use of colour and typefaces for medicine packs, to help differences to stand out.

Filik *et al.* (2006) found that use of 'tall man' letters to flag up differences in drug names that sound or look alike can be effective, provided the person is aware that is the purpose of the odd-looking mix of fonts.

In hospital (Roberts *et al.*, 2002) 14% of dispensing errors were attributed to mistakes in transcribing the medicine order from inpatient chart to pharmacy order sheet. This type of dispensing error is specific to hospital pharmacy practice. Recent studies have also mentioned errors when picking drug or patient names from computer menus.

Ashcroft found similar factors were reported to contribute to near misses and errors, although dispensing errors were considered more likely when the pharmacy was busier than normal. Both Ashcroft and Lynskey noted that pharmacists were more likely to make dispensing errors than technicians. This could reflect the fact that, in primary care, pharmacists do less dispensing and more checking than technicians. Spencer and Smith noted the reverse for hospital dispensing errors.

Error detection and checking routines

In the study by Savage *et al.*, 18 pharmacists completed a dispensing check under experimental conditions. All identified wrong drug or wrong strength errors, but eight missed a 'look-alike' patient name error.

Detecting a wrong patient name appeared to be more likely if reading the patient name was obviously part of the preparatory 'scoping' routine for the prescription. Four of the five people who did not read the name out loud missed the error on the dispensing label.

However, four people who did read the name out loud still failed to detect it was wrong on the label suggesting that a range of other error-producing factors (e.g. eyesight; type size; dyslexia) could also be involved.

It is widely held that checking by a second person is better than re-checking your own work, although experimental evidence to support this is limited. Bower (1990) analysed reports of near misses and dispensing errors made over a 6-month period

Table 3.4. Reported causes of dispensing errors

	Community[a]	Hospital[b]
Similar names	Yes	Yes
Similar packs	Yes	Yes
Stock in wrong place on shelf	Yes	Yes
Scrolling down drug list	Yes	Yes
Misreading prescription	Yes	Yes
Hard to read handwriting	Yes	Yes
Product or dose knowledge		Yes
Short of staff/new staff	Yes	Yes
Busyness	Yes	Yes
Interruptions	Yes	Yes
Tired/unwell/lack of focus		Yes

[a] Pharmacist reports (Ashcroft *et al.*, 2005; Lynskey *et al.*, 2007).
[b] Pharmacist reports and interview data (Spencer & Smith, 1993; Roberts & Spencer, 2002; Beso *et al.*, 2005).

in five hospitals using different final check routines. He suggested that dispensing errors were more likely with self-checking, but the total number of reports (119) was very low, with only 21 detected outside the dispensary. In Spencer and Smith's much larger (1993) study, 19 hospital pharmacies recorded data over 6 months; dispensing error rates were significantly higher in hospitals where technicians were checked, but pharmacists were not.

Ross *et al.* (2000) described a reduction in anonymous reports to a mandatory hospital medication error scheme after the pharmacy introduced the policy that two people should check all dispensing. But no system is foolproof: overall, authors noted that most (67% of 195) of all medication errors occurred despite 'second checking.'

Dispensing safely: the impact of new technologies

Product verification

The evidence set out above suggests that wrong drug or wrong strength errors are relatively common during the dispensing process, and that a small proportion of them escape the final dispensing check.

Wrong drug or wrong strength errors account for just under half of all errors reported to an unofficial hospital scheme (Roberts *et al.*, 2002). In Warner and Gerrett's community pharmacy study, a quarter of all dispensing mistakes (near misses and errors) concerned the wrong strength or wrong formulation of the drug. This ties in with reports to the NRLS, in which similar error patterns were seen in hospital and community reports.

Radio-frequency ID microchips or two-dimensional bar codes on medicine packs can be used to verify that the right product has been picked from the shelf. Interfaced with suitable visual display and other technology, these systems will also alert the pharmacist to out-of-date and counterfeit stock and allow product recalls. As Dean Franklin and O' Grady (2007) have pointed out, the effectiveness of such systems would improve if the scanning device was linked to the pharmacy records. In their study, such a system would have prevented around one in five of the moderately severe product picking errors. However, it would not have prevented the only severe error in this study; a labelling error involving doxycyline for malaria prophylaxis.

Robotic dispensing

Having a machine to do the picking is another option. There are two main types of automatic dispensing system; random storage, where dispensary stock is put away by the picking head, and channel storage, in which staff load stock manually into predetermined channels. The second type allows more stock to be stored in the same space, but could be more vulnerable to human error.

Slee *et al.* (2002) reported a 50% drop in internal dispensing errors (i.e. near misses detected by the dispensing check) in the first 4 months after introduction of their ROWA speedcase automated dispensing system. Fitzpatrick *et al.* (2005) found a smaller reduction of 16% with the Consis channel storage system.

This suggests differences between automated systems, and also that such systems can change the way that staff work. In Fitzpatrick's report, although the overall error rate went down, there was a 35% increase in 'wrong directions' labelling errors. The dispensing workload increased by 19%, but the average checking time remained the same, suggesting that the checking technicians were spending less time per prescription than they did before automation.

Automatic dispensing is expected to allow more efficient use of staff time, freeing up staff for clinical duties outside the dispensary.

The DoH has repeatedly emphasized the value of freeing up pharmacist time by delegating dispensing, or automating it (Audit Commission, 2001; DoH, 2004). In hospitals, this impacts on technicians and ATOs, rather than on pharmacists. In the community pharmacy, the aim is to cut technician time spent picking products, allowing them to take over labelling, so that pharmacists can spend more time with patients.

Rutter *et al.* (2001) evaluated the impact of an automated picking system linked to the dispensary computer using work sampling methods. Two pharmacists and three dispensers working in the same pharmacy were observed at work over defined time periods before and after introduction of the robot. The new system did not decrease time spent dispensing; the dispensing process on average took longer and became more labour-intensive for all. This suggests that staff need time to adapt to new technology, and also to adapt it to local prescribing patterns.

Automating product picking also did not give the pharmacists more time to spend with their patients. As others have found (Savage, 1995), time saved on dispensing can only be used for patient contact if the pharmacist's dispensing workload can be predicted in advance.

Electronic prescribing (EP)

Many healthcare workers believe that electronic prescribing (known as computerized physician order entry or CPOE in America) makes things safer because it improves legibility of medication orders (Kaushal & Bates, 2004; Barber *et al.*, 2006). Shulman *et al.* (2005) has demonstrated a significant reduction in prescribing errors after the introduction of CPOE in an intensive care unit. However, dispensing error rates with handwritten and computer-generated prescriptions have not been investigated.

The few UK hospitals that have EP all cite improved legibility and a reduction in prescription ambiguities (Goundrey Smith, 2006) as benefits. Having access to an electronic medication history, plus clinical notes and test results, helps pharmacists to manage an increasing clinical screening and dispensary workload to provide full clinical checking without having to make daily visits to wards (Barber *et al.*, 2006).

Most work on EP focuses on the reduction in prescribing and administration errors. Unpublished data from one hospital where staff levels have remained relatively constant for some years suggests that EP helps pharmacists manage an increasing clinical screening and dispensary workload (see Fig. 3.2). However, it does not help to reduce picking errors, and may initially increase labelling errors as staff adapt to new ways of working.

In primary care, a single electronic health record and the electronic transfer of prescriptions are key components of the NHS Connecting for Health programme. The potential benefits are that all pharmacists will have access to a complete medication

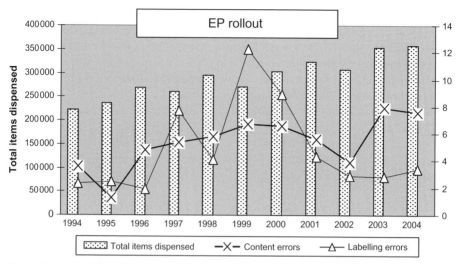

Figure 3.2. Annual dispensing volume and dispensing error rates in one district general hospital over 10 years. Electronic prescribing systems were introduced to wards between 1996 (care of the elderly) and 2002 (paediatrics). New versions of the software were introduced in June 1999 and again in May 2001.

record plus basic safety information such as drug allergies for the patient they are dispensing for.

GPs have prescribed electronically for years but the electronic transmission of these prescriptions (ETP) directly into pharmacy computers is only just starting. Most patients still present a paper 'token' prescription, from which their medication order can be read into the pharmacy computer by scanning a barcode. In the next phase of ETP roll-out, patients will be able to opt to have their prescriptions sent electronically to their nominated pharmacy. This will bring significant changes in dispensary checking practice, as the only prescription will be on a computer screen.

Implications for education and training

Dispensing is a core role for pharmacists. But, as the call for their traditional extemporaneous preparation skills has declined, and computer technology has advanced, the physical process of 'counting, pouring and sticking' has become a routine mundane activity which many pharmacists are keen to delegate to trained staff (Rutter, 2001). The increased emphasis on the clinical aspects of a pharmacist's job, particularly in hospital practice, the greater use of technicians and the view that machines are inherently safer than people are all contributing to a gradual downgrading of checking as a basic transferable skill, important for most types of work.

At undergraduate level, the emphasis is shifting away from practical dispensing and towards clinical prescription screening and medication management. Tutors may emphasize the importance of the pharmacist's role in patient safety, but students have limited opportunity to develop their basic skills.

This is of some concern as, according to human error theory (Reason, 1990), accuracy checking is a skill: a well-practised routine requiring little conscious thought. People who work in the dispensary infrequently may need more conscious effort to maintain this routine. Pharmacists who detected all the dispensing errors in Savage *et al.*'s checking experiment worked regularly and often in the dispensary and had well-established routines which were not compromised by distractions.

New technologies are already changing the way that dispensary staff work. Automated dispensing and product authentication systems may reduce certain types of dispensing error, but they may also make staff less careful.

Beso *et al.* (2005) have described a dispensary culture where errors are seen as being *'inevitable and sometimes acceptable'*, and in which there is a reliance on others to identify and rectify mistakes. These authors concluded that there is a need to explore ways to encourage all staff to take responsibility for dispensing and labelling. The best place for this to start is during the pharmacy undergraduate course.

References

Ashcroft DM, Quinlan P, Blenkinsopp A. (2005). Prospective study of the incidence, nature and causes of dispensing errors in community pharmacies. *Pharmacoepidemiology and Drug Safety*, **14**, 327–32.

Audit Commission. (Dec 2001). *A Spoonful of Sugar – Medicines Management in NHS Hospitals*. London: Audit Commission.

Barber N, Dean Franklin B, Cornford T, Klecun E, Savage I. (2006). Safer, faster, better? Evaluating electronic prescribing. Report for the Patient Safety Research Programme, Department of Health. Published at: http://pcpoh.bham.ac.uk/publichealth/psrp/Publication_PS019.htm

Batty R, Barber N. (1992). Ward pharmacy: a foundation for prescribing audit? *Quality in Health Care*, **1**, 5–9.

Bellingham C. (2004). What the new contract has in store. *Pharmaceutical Journal*, **273**, 385.

Beso A, Dean Franklin B, Barber N. (2005). The frequency and potential causes of dispensing errors in a hospital pharmacy. *Pharmacy World and Science*, **27**, 182–90.

Bower AC. (1990). Dispensing error rates in hospital pharmacy. *Pharmaceutical Journal* (suppl. Feb 17), **244**, R22–3.

Chen YF, Neil KE, Avery AJ, Dewey ME, Johnson C. (2005). Prescribing errors and other problems reported by community pharmacists. *Journal of Therapeutics and Clinical Risk Management*, **1**(4), 333–42.

Dean Franklin B, O'Grady K, Donyai P, Jacklin A, Barber N. (2007). The impact of a closed loop electronic prescribing and automated dispensing system on the ward pharmacist's time and activities. *International Journal of Pharmacy Practice*, **15**, 133–9.

Dean Franklin B, O'Grady K. (2007). Dispensing errors in community pharmacy: frequency, clinical significance and potential impact of authentication at the point of dispensing. *International Journal of Pharmacy Practice*, **15**, 273–81.

Department of Health. (2004). *Building a Safer NHS for Patients – Improving Medication Safety*. London: HMSO.

Edmondson H, Chua SS, Lee PC, Wong ICK. (2003). A preliminary study of a dispensing error reporting scheme for primary care pharmacists in Hull and East Riding. *Pharmacy World and Science*, **25**, A26–7.

Filik R, Purdy K, Gale A, Garrett D. (2006). Labelling of medicines and patient safety: evaluating methods of reducing drug name confusion. *Human Factors*, **48**(1), 39–47.

Fitzpatrick R, Cooke P, Southall C, Kauldhar K, Waters P. (2005). Evaluation of an automated dispensing system in a hospital pharmacy dispensary.

Pharmaceutical Journal, **274**, 763–5.

Goundrey-Smith S. (2006). Electronic prescribing-experience in the UK and system design issues. *Pharmaceutical Journal,* **277**, 485–9.

Greene R. (1995). Survey of prescription anomalies in community pharmacies. *Pharmaceutical Journal,* **254**, 476–81, 873–5.

Hawkey C, Hodgson S, Norman A, Daneshmend T, Garner S. (1990). Effect of reactive pharmacy intervention on quality of hospital prescribing. *British Medical Journal,* **300**, 986–90.

Kaushal R, Bates DW. (2002). Information technology and medication safety: what is the benefit? *Quality and Safety in Health Care,* **11**, 261–5.

Lynskey D, Haigh SJ, Patel N, Macadam AB. (2007). Medication errors in community pharmacy: an investigation into the types and causes. *International Journal of Pharmacy Practice,* **15**, 105–12.

National Patient Safety Agency. (2007). *Safety in Doses: 4th Report from the Patient Safety Observatory.* London: NPSA.

Nemeth C, Cook R. (2005). Hiding in plain sight: What Koppel *et al.* tell us about healthcare IT. *Journal of Biomedical Informatics,* **38**, 262–3.

Reason J. (1990). *Human Error.* Cambridge: Cambridge University Press.

Roberts DE, Spencer MG, Burfield R, Bowden S. (2002). An analysis of dispensing errors in NHS hospitals. *International Journal of Pharmacy Practice,* **10**(suppl), R6.

Ross LM, Wallace J, Paton JY. (2000). Medication errors in a paediatric teaching hospital in the UK: five years operational experience. *Archives of Disease in Childhood,* **83**, 492–7.

Royal Pharmaceutical Society of Great Britain. (July 2007). *Medicines, Ethics and Practice.* London: RPSGB, p. 98.

Rutter PM, Brown D, Portlock JC. (2001). Can automated dispensing decrease prescription turn-around time and alter staff work patterns? *International Journal of Pharmacy Practice,* **9**(suppl), R22.

Savage I. (1995). Time for customer contact in pharmacies with and without a dispensing technician. *International Journal of Pharmacy Practice,* **3**, 193–9.

Savage I. (1999). The changing face of pharmacy practice – evidence from 20 years of work sampling studies. *International Journal of Pharmacy Practice,* **7**(4), 209–19.

Savage I, Bissenden B, Martin C. (2007). *Learning to Teach the Final Check.* London: Pharmacy Practice Research Trust.

Shah S, Aslam M, Avery A. (2001). A survey of prescription errors in general practice. *Pharmaceutical Journal,* **267**, 860–2.

Shulman JI, Shulman S, Haines AP. (1981). The prevention of adverse drug reactions – a potential role for pharmacists in the primary health team? *Journal of the Royal College of General Practice,* **31**, 429–34.

Shulman R, Singer M, Goldstone J, Bellingan G. (2005). Medication errors: a prospective cohort study of hand-written and computerised physician order entry in the intensive care unit. *Clinical Care,* **9**, R516–21.

Slee A, Farrar K, Hughes D. 2002. Implementing an automated dispensing system. *Pharmaceutical Journal,* **268**, 437–8.

Spencer MG, Smith AP. (1993). A multicentre study of dispensing errors in British hospitals. *International Journal of Pharmacy Practice,* **2**, 142–6.

Stevens RG, Balon D. (1997). Detection of hazardous drug–drug interactions in a community pharmacy and subsequent intervention. *International Journal of Pharmacy Practice,* **5**, 142–8.

Stubbs J, Haw C, Cahill C. (2004). Auditing prescribing errors in a psychiatric hospital. Are pharmacists' interventions effective? *Hospital Pharmacist*, **11**, 203–6.

Tuthill A, Wood K, Cavell G. 2004. Audit of drug allergy documentation on inpatient charts. *Pharmacy World and Science*, **26**, a48–9.

Warner B, Gerrett D. (2005). Identification of medication error through community pharmacies. *International Journal of Pharmacy Practice*, **13**, 223–8.

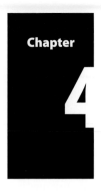

Chapter

4

Safety in administering

Jane Watson and Liz Plastow

Administration of a medication can be defined as 'the giving by a nurse or authorised person of a drug to a patient'.
(Anderson & Anderson, 1995)

Background

In the United Kingdom it is estimated that 2 500 000 medicines are prescribed for use within hospitals and the community setting every day (DH, 2004). Reports from the National Prescribing Centre (NPC, 2007) suggest that 15% of health expenditure is spent on prescribed medicines and this is the most common form of medicinal intervention.

Definition

A prescribed medicinal product is usually referred to simply as a medicine and for the purpose of this chapter a medicinal product will be referred to simply as a 'medicine'.

The definition of a medicinal product is:

'Any substance or combination of substances presented as having properties for treating or preventing disease in human beings.'

'Any substance or combination of substances which may be used in or administered to human beings either with a view to restoring, correcting or modifying physiological functions by exerting a pharmacological, immunological or metabolic action, or to making a medical diagnosis' (MHRA, 2007).

Medicinal products come in a variety of formulations. They may include: tablets, capsules, liquids, elixirs, syrups, pastilles, lozenges, mixtures, drops, creams, ointments, lotions, parenteral infusion, inhalations, sprays, transdermal patches, pessaries, rectal preparations, e.g. suppositories, enemas and also medication may be given by an injectable route. This is by no means an exhaustive list, but what is important is that, whenever a medical formulation is used, basic principles must be followed to ensure the safe administration of that product.

Medicines Management has been defined as 'A system of processes and behaviours that determine how medicines are used by patients and the NHS' (Alexander *et al.*, 2004). In order to be effective medicines, management puts the patient at the centre of care, patients are better informed and care is targeted at the point of delivery through maximizing the use of resources and making better use of professional skills and knowledge. By appropriately managing the safe administration of medicines, nurses are key to improving patient satisfaction and reducing unwanted effects of medication and preventing hospital admissions. It has been suggested that preventable adverse reactions to medicines are implicated in up to 17% of hospital admissions in older patients;

Medication Safety: An Essential Guide, ed. Molly Courtenay and Matt Griffiths. Published by Cambridge University Press. © M. Courtenay and M. Griffiths 2009.

in addition, whilst in hospital a further 17% of older patients will suffer an adverse drug reaction during their stay (DH, 2001). Healthcare professionals should be aware when patients are taking a number of medications that this may further increase the risk of adverse reactions, which may result in increased risk of admission to hospital, and when considering care to the patient not only should they consider each individual medication but also possible interactions between medicines. Research indicates that as many as 50% of patients do not take their medication as prescribed (RPSGB & Merck, Sharp and Dohme, 1997); it should therefore never be assumed, just because medication is prescribed, that it has been taken as indicated. Lack of adherence to medicine regimes can be an issue for hospitalized patients and it is therefore important to apply the principles of medicines management to address inappropriate and ineffective use of medicines at all times.

Self-administration

The majority of individuals for whom a medicine is prescribed will be able to self-administer in accordance with the instructions provided by the prescriber. Most self-administration occurs in the home setting and is accepted as everyday practice, by both the patient and the prescriber. Where this is not possible, there are a number of people who may be available to help and support medicine taking. A health or social care worker may be involved but, in many instances, it is the family member, friend or neighbour who may assist in the administration of a medicine. Where a healthcare professional has responsibility for the patient, it is essential that they assess the suitability of the care giver to administer medicines, and if there is any cause for concern, he/she has a duty to act accordingly, either by assisting the care giver and ensuring competence and safety or in informing colleagues to ensure a more appropriate package of care is available for the patient. It should never be assumed that, just because the patient is in their own home and being cared for, the carer understands how to give medication, its purpose, side effects and anticipated outcome.

Concordance with medication is a major issue and many people will stop taking medication if they do not feel it to be beneficial or if they experience side effects. However, with appropriate education about their medicines, concordance can be significantly increased. A lack of adherence to treatment regimes is not just about forgetting medicines, it may be a choice by the patient based on beliefs and factors that are individually important to them. However, motivation to take medicines may be increased where the patient understands and accepts their diagnosis, they agree with the medicines prescribed and have had the opportunity to express their concerns specifically and they feel these have been fully addressed (Medicines Partnership, 2004).

Information for patients about their medicines is available from a number of possible sources. These include patient information leaflets (found in all dispensed medication), clinical knowledge summaries, patient leaflets, NHS Direct On-line, NHS Choices and Patient UK (Patient UK). As a healthcare professional, you should consider the patient holistically and, where necessary, you may need to provide information in a number of formats, e.g. audiotapes, videos, leaflets in different languages or Braille.

In hospitals and other care settings, self-administration is not always an option, although in recent years there have been changes to practice, so as to encourage independence, which have resulted in increased opportunities for patients in hospitals to self-administer their medication. Within the hospital or care setting it is important that registrants assess a patient as to their suitability to self-administer and that, in doing so, they work within both professional and organizational guidelines. There must be assurance that the patient will take the medication as prescribed and that there is no risk to other patients in accessing medication which is not prescribed for them. It should be recognized that patients will not necessarily consider the risk to other patients if they leave medication by their bed or do not lock their medicines away. When patients choose to self-administer, this provides an opportunity for health professionals to both assess the patient's ability to 'take' their medication as prescribed, but also to establish their understanding of the prescribed medication, which supports the principle of concordance (NPC, 2007). An additional benefit is the potential to reduce the risk of medication errors, especially in respect to the wrong medication being given to a named patient.

Where a patient's condition does not permit the self-administration of a medicine in a hospital or alternative care setting, the administration of a medicine must be undertaken by a healthcare care practitioner or other authorized person.

Duty of care

Health professionals have a duty of care to patients and this includes all aspects related to the administration of medication. They must be able to justify their decision-making and must work within professional codes of conduct (NMC, 2008; RSPGB, 2007). Staff who undertake the administration must ensure they follow the guidelines and standards for this task set by their employer. Failure to do so could result in the employer's vicarious liability not being upheld.

Where patients ask a third person to help with the administration of their medicine, it is the responsibility of the health professional to ensure that the directions as laid down by the prescriber have been understood. It is the patient's right to determine who will administer the medication; however, the prescriber and/or health professional involved in the patient's care has a duty to ensure that any information required to ensure the safe administration of the medicine is provided and understood. Failure to do so could result in harm and if a patient decides to take legal action, the health professional's practice could be brought into question.

In spite of both professional and organizational standards, it is concerning that the number of medication errors remain significant in the UK; in fact medication errors are the most common reason for referral to the Nursing and Midwifery Council, the regulatory body for nurses, midwives and specialist community public health nurses. Nonetheless, there are numerous medications administered or self-administered daily without incident.

Medication errors

The National Patient Safety Agency (NPSA) reported 60 000 medication incidents, in an 18-month period from January 2005 to June 2006. Ninety-two of the incidents reported resulted in severe harm or death to the patient. The impact of medication error may lead to severe consequences for the patient and their family and also to the healthcare professional and employing organization.

In addition to the significant consequences for the patient and their family, medication error could result in action by the employer, the professional regulatory body, and in criminal and /or civil prosecution. It is not unknown, where medication errors have occurred, for the employer to suspend a healthcare professional and to make a referral to the regulatory body who may investigate and take necessary action. In addition, because the administration of medicines is regulated by legislation, if the action were a breach of medicines legislation, a criminal case could be taken, and a civil prosecution made by the patient and their family. Healthcare professionals should never underestimate their responsibility when administering medication or choosing to omit it.

The National Patient Safety Agency has identified trends in medication errors and they fall into four main categories:

- The incorrect medicine being selected for administration.
- The incorrect dose being administered.
- The incorrect strength of the medication being administered.
- The prescribed/dispensed medication being omitted.

In response to the identified themes in medication administration errors, the NPSA have put systems in place to reduce these errors and the subsequent consequences for all involved in the process. All healthcare professionals should be familiar with the Drug Alerts published by the NPSA and ensure they receive information on all national documents that are published. Where a medicines management or pharmaceutical advisor is employed by their Trust they should familiarize themselves with that person and ensure they are on all circulation lists, to ensure they receive all information and keep themselves as up to date as possible.

Standards for Medicines Management

The Nursing and Midwifery Council (NMC) set out the regulatory requirements for the safe administration of medicines:-

'When required to administer medication a practitioner is accountable for his or her own actions and omissions. The practitioner must satisfy himself or herself, they have the necessary information to ensure the safe administration of the medicine. This will include access to the patient's record in addition to information about the medicine to be administered' (NMC, 2007).

In addition, the NMC have developed basic principles that should be followed, which will promote safe and appropriate administration of a medicine.

Authorization to administer

The first step in the safe administration of medicines is the 'authorization' to administer. Practitioners will often refer to the prescription as being the authorization. This is not technically true: the prescription which must be signed by a prescriber (it may be any registered independent and/or supplementary prescriber – it does not need to be a medical prescriber) gives authority to a pharmacist (or other) to dispense the medication, it does not give the healthcare professional the authority to administer.

Prior to the administration of a medicinal product the health professional must have access to one of the following for authorization for the administration of the medicines or medicines:

- Patient Specific Direction, which can include a Patient Medicines Administration Chart (often referred to as a MAR Chart).
- Patient Group Direction, which the registered practitioner has signed as competent to operate under the identified direction.

Or if:

- As a professional they are working within 'Medicines Exemption' Prescription Only Medicines (Human Use Order) 1997 SI No. 1830 (the POM Order); Medicines (Pharmacy and General sales Exemption) Order 1980 SI No. 1924 and Medicines (Sale or Supply) (Miscellaneous Provisions) Regulations 1980 SI No. 1923 in accordance with their professional practice or
- Working within an agreed list identified by the employer of 'General Sales List Medicines'.

A Patient Specific Direction (PSD) including a patient medicines administration chart

These forms will identify the individual patient for which a named drug or drugs are to be administered. They have to be signed by a registered prescriber and will include the following:

- The name of the patient to which the prescribed medication/s is to be administered.
- Other forms of individual patient identification. These may include one or more of the following;

NHS Number
Date of Birth
Hospital Number
Address

The Patient Specific Direction must include:
The name of the medicinal product to be used and its strength.
The dose to be used.
The formulation to be used.
The route of administration.
The frequency of administration.
The duration of the treatment regime.
Any specific instructions, e.g. before food.

The prescriber must sign the direction to administer.

Patient Group Direction (PGD)

A Patient Group Direction is a written instruction for the supply or the administration of a named licence medicine for an individual who is not individually identified before presentation, to enable staff to administer a medication under a PGD legislation. This was introduced as outlined in the Health Service Circular 2000/026 (DH, 2006); similar guidance is in place in Wales, Northern Ireland and Scotland.

Patient Group Directions are developed locally and the HSC 2000/026 outlines the organizations that can develop PGDs and the criteria of staff that can operate under them.

Healthcare professionals are required to sign PGDs in order to permit them to administer the medication that is named in each separate direction. In signing the PGD, staff are signing to state that they are competent to determine the medication that is required and that they are competent to administer it. The National Prescribing Centre (NPC), a practical guide and framework of competencies for all professionals using patient group directions (NPC 2004), details the competencies required to administer medication under a patient group direction. It is recommended that all healthcare professionals using a PGD, as part of their continuing professional development, access this framework and identify their level of competence, not just assume they are 'competent'. Patient Group Directions are relatively new and there are a number of senior professionals who are very experienced but may not fully understand their accountability and responsibility in supplying and administering medication under a PGD.

In operating under a PGD the registered practitioner must take a comprehensive history to ensure that the patient identified does not meet any of the exclusion criteria. If this were to be the case they should neither supply nor administer medication to that patient.

The legislation specifies the professional groups that can operate under a PGD. These include currently nurses, midwives, specialist community public health nurses, paramedics, optometrists, pharmacists, orthotists, chiropodists, radiographers, physiotherapists, dieticians, occupational therapists, speech and language therapists and prosthetists, but does not include student nurses. Student nurses and midwives may administer medication under supervision, but not take responsibility for administration under a PGD. Since September 2007, the Nursing and Midwifery Council have mandated that all pre-registration courses will require students successfully to meet the competencies required to operate under a PGD.

It should be noted that, when using a PGD, the eligible healthcare professional who supplies the medication *must* also be the healthcare professional who administers it. Under current medicines legislation it is illegal to delegate to any third party even if they are a qualified practitioner.

Medicines exemptions

There are three main groups entitled to supply and administer medication under the Medicines Exemptions. These are paramedics, midwives and occupational health nurses. The exemptions do not allow paramedics, midwives and nurses to *prescribe*; they give them the authority to administer certain drugs, in given situations that have been identified within a list of authorized medications. There must be a written instruction within a policy that enables the administration. The legislation that enables exemptions are Prescription Only Medicines (Human Use Order) 1997 SI No. 1830 (the POM Order); Medicines (Pharmacy and General Sales Exemption) Order 1980 SI No. 1924 and Medicines (Sale or Supply) (Miscellaneous Provisions) Regulations 1980 SI No. 1923Act. This entitles the individual to supply and administer medicines from an exempted list without an individual written instruction.

Homely medicines

Organizations may agree a list of medications which can be administered by clinicians, where there is no patient-specific direction or patient group direction and where medicines exemptions do not apply. These medicines are often referred to as homely or discretionary medicines; it should be noted, however, that strict conditions apply. The *only* medicines that may be administered in this way are General Sales List (GSL) and Pharmacy Only (P) medicines. On *no* account must a Prescription Only Medicine (POM) or a Controlled Drug (CD) be administered in this way; this would be illegal and could lead to prosecution. There must also be organizational protocols in place, with clear instructions on the administration of these homely remedies/discretionary medicines. The instructions should include: the name of the medicinal product to be administered, the dose, the frequency and the time limitation before referral to a medical practitioner.

Staff working between, or transferring from, organizations must check the local protocols/guidelines prior to administering a medication under a discretionary medicines list.

The first principle in the administration of a medication is the 'authority' to administer and identification of the appropriate authority for the clinical situation you are working in.

If you are administering a medication and you are unsure of the instructions contained within the authority to administer, it is the duty of the administering person to check the details with the prescriber. Whenever a registrant comes across a new drug in practice, it would be expected that further information be sought routinely to ensure the registrant clearly understands the pharmaco-therapeutic effect of the drug and its indications. Additional information on the medicines prescribed include dose range, side effects, contraindications and drug interactions, which can be accessed from documents such as the British National Formulary (BNF) or in the summary of product characteristics (SPC). The SPC are available through the manufacturer or via the website www.medicines.org.uk.

As a registrant you should have sufficient knowledge of the pharmaceutical product you are administering; this should be at a level such that you are able to question any uncertainty in the dose, route of administration, frequency and potential interaction with other medicines being taken. In addition, the registrant or delegated administrator must have an underlying knowledge of the medical condition for which the medication is being administered.

As a practitioner you have the right (and duty) to question any part of the authorization to administer a medication if unclear about the instruction or the preparation. Although this may seem daunting, especially if you are a student nurse or early in your career, safety of the patient is paramount and this may mean you need to challenge a senior colleague. Be prepared though to be challenged back and be clear what it is you're questioning. If it is your own understanding, make that clear; if it's because your knowledge, skills and competence tells you that something is wrong – don't be afraid to challenge.

Allergy status

Ensuring a patient's allergy status has been identified and recorded is essential for all patients and, if there is no allergy status recorded, it should be ascertained as a matter of course. This is a key requirement in helping to reduce medication errors and potentially the death of a patient. At all stages of the administration this should be checked. There may be local policies in place to identify an individual's allergy to a medicinal product. When working in an area, the registrant must make themselves aware of local procedures. If the means of identifying allergy status is not apparent, then it may be appropriate to raise this and suggest greater importance is given to alerting all staff when a patient has an allergy and a policy is in place to address this. Although it is deemed 'best practice', not all medications will be prescribed using the generic name; on occasions a 'brand name' may be used. It is therefore important when a patient states they are allergic to a medicine that you check the 'brand names' as well, to avoid inadvertent administration. You should, however, always be aware that a patient may present with a previously unknown allergic reaction to a medication, and so be sure that you follow policy and know what to do.

Allergies can present in a number of ways. An allergic response is not always an anaphylactic one; a mild, moderate or severe rash that appears within a short period (24–78 hours) following administration may indicate a reaction to a medicine. Whatever response is noted, you should discuss with a senior member of staff, and any significant reaction/response should be notified to the Medicines Healthcare Products Regulatory Authority (www.MHRA.org) through the Yellow Card Scheme.

Administration of medication

Having identified the appropriate authority to administer a medication, and that the patient has no allergies, the following steps must be followed to ensure safe administration.

You must check each step of the process:

Check that you have the correct patient.

The National Patient Safety Agency 2004 in their framework for action 'Right patient–right care' (NPSA, 2004) outlines methods of correctly identifying patients and these methods include the following:

- Check the name of the patient against the documentation giving authority to administer or the patient's notes, if operating under a PGD 'Medicines Exemption' or local protocols.
- Ask the patient their name.
- Check the patient's identity against the identification bracelet if worn. As this would not be possible within the patient's home environment, it is important to remember there should not be an assumption made that the person who opens the door or whom you are talking to is the patient.
- In certain circumstances and having gained consent (DH, 2001), it may be necessary to ascertain identity, using a photograph. When using photographic identity, it is important to have a process in place to update the photograph on a regular basis. In addition, when obtaining consent, there must be local policies in place, which include consideration of the patient's mental capacity to give informed consent.
- Where identification through asking the patient, via a name bracelet or a photograph, is not possible or practical, the service must have identified other

methods of determining identification. If you are not sure, you should always seek information from your medicines management lead, nursing or pharmacy lead.

As with all procedures, gaining the patient's consent to administer is essential (DH, 2001; NMC, 2007). There will be certain circumstances where gaining verbal or written consent is not possible, e.g. the unconscious patient; however, you should ensure you are aware of the local arrangements and policies that are in place. Failure to do so and administering medication without consent and not following employer's policies could find you acting outside of vicarious liability. This is particularly important when medication is administered in a life-threatening situation. Where failure to administer could result in harm, being aware of local policy is essential. For patients who cannot give consent due to mental health difficulties, the issue is addressed in the Mental Capacity Act 2005, with which you should familiarize yourself.

There will be occasions where consent for the administration of medicines will be obtained by the person with parental responsibility. The Department of Health 2001 guidelines on consent will outline this process and organizations should have policies in place as to how this will be documented.

Ensure that the patient is ready to receive the medication.

This is particularly relevant when the medication has to be prepared prior to administration. Medication should not be prepared in advance and left for the patient to take or for another professional to administer (NMC, 2007).

Check that, prior to preparing the medication, you have all the equipment required and if appropriate, training in the use of that equipment to undertake the task.

Check the medication. The following checks must be made against the authority to administer and the medicinal product itself and this must take place each time you administer medication in any format.

1. Check the name of the medication to ensure the correct drug is going to be administered. This will involve checking the name on the dispensed container and if the drug is contained within a container, e.g. an ampoule, making an additional check on removing the preparation from its original container.
2. Check that the right formulation of the drug is available.
3. Check the strength of the preparation that is going to be administered.
4. Check that the right dose of the drug is to be administered.
5. Check that the formulation available is suitable for the route of administration authorized.
6. Check the frequency of administration. At this point it is essential to check against patient's records for the time of the last administration to ensure it has not already been given within the time scale.
7. Check the expiry date of the medicine.
8. Visibly check the product (where appropriate) for any contamination.

On occasions, a drug calculation may be required. If a calculation is required, this should be documented and retained within the patient's notes. For complex calculations, it may be appropriate for a second person to undertake the calculation independently and compare the results. If there are discrepancies in the calculations, then the prescriber or lead clinician should be contacted. If in doubt over a calculation, always check with a colleague; it is a sign of professional responsibility to do so, not a weakness.

Check the route of administration against the authorization to administer or the details within the PGD.

Check that, if you are administering a medicine, that you are aware of the technique for administration and do not undertake the task if the technique to be used is outside your area of competence.

Check that the patient's allergy status has been recorded and it would be considered good practice to ask the patient again, if appropriate, of any known allergies.

You must delay an administration if you are unsure of the clinical condition of the patient in relation to the drug you are administering. This refers both to allergy status and possible changes to the individual's clinical condition. For example, when administering digoxin, if the pulse is below 60 beats per minute, it should not be given and the action taken should be documented, including the patient's pulse.

If you are questioning at any point the administration of a medicine, in relation to the authority to administer, the drug, dose, route of administration, or potential drug interaction, the prescriber must be contacted. The outcome of the conversation must be documented in accordance with national guidelines and employer policy on record keeping.

Extra caution should be taken in the administration of controlled drugs. There are additional guidelines relating to the administration of controlled drugs, these are outlined in *Safer Management of Controlled Drugs: A Guide to Good Practice in Secondary Care* (England) (DoH, 2007b) and *Safer Management of Controlled Drugs: Monitoring and Inspection Guidelines – Core Activities for Controlled Drug Monitoring and Inspection Work in Primary Care* (RPSGB & DH, 2006).

The above requirements are the basic principles that should be adhered to in the administration of any medicinal product in any format. In addition to the basic principles for administration of medication, there are occasions when additional checks should be undertaken.

A second signature is required when administering a controlled drug in a secondary care or equivalent setting. The second signatory should make the required checks against the authorization sheet and is responsible for these checks. If at any stage of the procedure the second signatory is not sure of the details, they must not sign as a second signatory. The second signatory will also be responsible for checking any drug calculation that is relevant to the administration of the controlled drug. It is considered best practice that the second person should witness the whole administration process.

One area where it is not always possible to obtain a second signature is the patient's home environment. The controlled drug will have been prescribed and subsequently dispensed by a pharmacist. It is suggested that the second signature requirements should be based on local risk assessment; however, if practical, a second person should undertake the checking process. The NMC have indicated that it would be considered acceptable, if a healthcare professional was not available to undertake the second check, for a responsible competent person to do so. This could be the patient or a responsible carer (NMC, 2007).

Delegation of administration of medicines

There are occasions where the registered practitioner will be required to delegate the administration of the medicine to another person. Accountability for delegation always remains with the registered practitioner unless delegated to another registered practitioner, who would, by accepting to administer, then accept professional responsibility for their actions. The most important aspect of delegation to a junior member of staff is that the professional delegating ensures the person to whom they have delegated the task is competent to do so. If the person accepting the delegated task is a qualified practitioner, they must understand that they are also accepting accountability to undertake the administration and must act in accordance with NMC standards and local policies.

Competencies may be defined as 'a quality or characteristic of a person which is related to effective or superior performance'. Competencies can be described as knowledge skills, motives and personal traits (NPC, 2000). The development of a competency framework is designed to ensure that whoever delivers a service, and wherever a patient may be seen, they will receive, at all times, high-quality interventions. Competencies may be further divided into task-based competencies and behavioural ones.

In delegating administration of medication, you must ensure you have given the necessary information to ensure safe administration including giving information on the drug, dose, strength and method/technique of administration. You must also ensure the person to whom you are delegating is competent with the technique and with any equipment that should be used, as well as the underpinning knowledge of the drug and clinical condition of the patient. It is often the latter issues, the knowledge of the drug and the clinical condition of the patient, that are overlooked and yet would be the areas on which any prosecuting barrister would focus their cross-examination on, should harm be the result of medicines administration.

You should never assume that, because someone has delegated the administration to you, they have assessed the clinical condition of the patient and that they themselves have understood the pharmaco-therapeutic action of the medication.

There will be instances where the delegation to administer the medication will be to a non-professional, e.g. a parent, family member or friend. In this case, when delegating the administration, you as the registrant retain accountability. You must ensure the person who has accepted the delegated task has the appropriate knowledge to complete the task safely, the competencies to do so, and is willing to accept the responsibility for their actions.

However, it must be remembered that you *cannot* delegate the administration of a medication if you are operating under a Patient Group Direction. The HSC 2000/026 states that the registered practitioner can only administer under a PGD if they have assessed the patient and signed to operate under the relevant PGD to administer the medication. Under a PGD, if you supply the medication, you must also administer the medication. It is currently illegal to delegate to another registered practitioner to give it. If you have supplied the drug to a patient and he/she wishes to administer it at a later date, only the healthcare professional who supplied the drug may administer it, but the patient himself can administer it for it is his 'property' because it has been supplied to him.

If an individual patient chooses to delegate the administration of a medicine to a third party, that is their choice; however, healthcare professionals still retain a duty to provide advice and support concerning administration.

Having obtained the necessary authority to administer the medication and been satisfied that the right medicine is to be given to the right patient, who has given consent, the next step is to prepare the medication.

Preparing medication prior to administration

All medication should be prepared in line with the recommendations from the manufacturers. Instruction on the preparation of a medicine is included in all dispensed preparations. Further instructions can be obtained from the summary of product characteristics (found in all dispensed medicines) and the British National Formulary. Having checked the summary of product characteristics and the directions on the dispensed medication, there are a number of additional precautions that you should consider:

- Tablets should not be handled, as the contamination may alter the coating of the medication.
- Tablets should not be crushed unless this has been identified as a suitable method of administration of the medicine.
- Capsules should not be split unless it has been identified as a suitable method to administer the medication.
- If liquid medications are being administered and a syringe is being used, the correct equipment should be used as identified by the National Patient Safety Agency *Alert 19*.

The National Patient Safety Agency has highlighted the administration of medicines intravenously as an area of high concern with respect to patient safety and, in response, has published the National Patient Safety Agency (-NPSA-)*Alert 20* (2007), which provides further guidance when preparing a medicine for injection.

Withdrawing solution from an ampoule (glass or plastic) into a syringe

Tap the ampoule gently to dislodge any medicine in the neck.

Snap open the neck of the ampoule taking care, if the ampoule is glass, that it does not shatter.

Attach a needle to a syringe and draw the required volume of solution into the syringe. Tilt the ampoule if necessary.

Invert the syringe and tap lightly to aggregate the air bubbles at the needle end. Expel air with care.

Remove the needle from the syringe and fit new needle or sterile blind hub.

Label the syringe if appropriate.

Keep the ampoule and any unused medicine until the administration to the patient is complete. This enables further checking to be undertaken if required.

If the ampoule contains a suspension rather than a solution, it should be gently swirled to mix the contents immediately before they are drawn into the syringe.

The neck of some plastic ampoules is designed to connect directly to a syringe without the use of a needle, after the top of the ampoule has been twisted off.

Withdrawing a solution or suspension from a vial into a syringe

Remove the tamper-evident seal from the vial and wipe the rubber septum with an alcohol wipe. Allow drying for at least 30 seconds.

With the needle sheathed, draw into the syringe a volume of air equivalent to the required volume of solution to be drawn up.

Remove the needle cover and insert the needle into the vial through the rubber septum.

Invert the vial. Keep the needle in the solution and slowly depress the plunger to push the air into the vial.

Release the plunger so that the solution flows back into the syringe.

If a large volume of solution is to be withdrawn, use a push–pull technique. Repeatedly inject small volumes of air and draw up an equal volume of solution until the required total is reached. This 'equilibrium method', i.e. equal volumes of air and solution, helps to minimize the build up of pressure in the vial.

Alternatively, the rubber septum can be pierced with a second needle to let air into the vial as solution is withdrawn. The tip of the vent needle must always be kept above the solution to prevent leakage.

With the vial still attached, invert the syringe. With the needle and vial uppermost, tap the syringe lightly to aggregate the bubbles at the end of the needle end. Push the air back into the vial.

Fill the syringe with the required volume and in accordance with the dose prescribed.

Remove the needle from the syringe and fit a new needle or sterile blind hub.

Label the syringe if appropriate.

Keep the vial and any unused medicine until the administration to the patient is complete. This enables further checking to be undertaken if required.

If the vial contains a suspension rather than a solution, it should be gently swirled to mix the contents immediately before they are drawn into the syringe.

Reconstituting powder in a vial and drawing the resulting solution or suspension into a syringe

Remove the tamper-evident seal from the vial and wipe the rubber septum with an alcohol wipe. Allow drying for at least 30 seconds.

Check the prescribed diluents for the reconstitute and the volume required.

Inject the diluents into the vial. Keeping the tip of the needle above the level of the solution in the vial, release the plunger. The syringe will fill with the air that has been displaced by the solution (if the contents of the vial were packed under a vacuum, solution will be drawn into the vial and no air will be displaced). If a large volume of diluents is to be added, use a push–pull technique.

With the syringe and needle still in place, gently swirl the vials(s) to dissolve all the powder, unless otherwise indicated by the product information. This may take several minutes.

With the needle sheathed, draw into the syringe a volume of air equivalent to the required volume of solution to be drawn up.

Remove the needle cover and insert the needle into the vial through the rubber septum.

Invert the vial. Keep the needle in the solution and slowly depress the plunger to push the air into the vial.

Release the plunger so that the solution flows back into the syringe.

If a large volume of solution is to be withdrawn, use a push–pull technique. Repeatedly inject small volumes of air and draw up an equal volume of solution until the required total is reached. The 'equilibrium method' helps to minimize the build-up of pressure in the vial.

Alternatively, the rubber septum can be pierced with a second needle to let air into the vial as the solution is withdrawn. The tip of the vent must always be kept above the solution to prevent leakage.

With the vial still attached, invert the syringe. With the needle and vial uppermost, tap the syringe lightly to aggregate the bubbles at the end of the needle end. Push the air back into the vial.

Fill the syringe with the required volume and in accordance with the dose pre-scribed.

Remove the needle from the syringe and fit a new needle or sterile blind hub.

Label the syringe if appropriate.

Keep the vial and any unused medicine until the administration to the patient is complete. This enables further checking to be undertaken if required.

If a purpose-designed reconstitution device is used, the manufacturer's instructions should be read carefully and followed closely. If you are too familiar with the device, additional training must be undertaken and competencies assessed.

Adding a medication to an infusion

Check that the infusion solution to which the medication is to be added is the prescribed fluid.

Check the medication to be added against the prescription chart.

Prepare the medicine as described in the sections above.

Check the outer wrapper of the infusion container for any signs of damage.

Check the wrapper and check the infusion container itself in good light. It should be intact and show no evidence of leaks or punctures.

Visibly check the solution, check the solution is not 'hazy' and is free from particles and/or discolouration.

Where necessary, remove the tamper-evident seal on the additive port according to the manufacturer's instructions, or wipe the rubber septum on the infusion container with an alcohol wipe, and allow drying for at least 30 seconds.

If the volume of medicine solution to be added is more than 10% of the initial contents of the infusion container (more than 50 ml to a 500 ml or 100 ml to a 1 litre infusion), an equivalent volume must first be removed with a syringe and needle.

Inject the medicine into the infusion container through the centre of the injection port, taking care to keep the tip of the needle away from the side of the infusion container. Withdraw the needle and invert the container at least five times to ensure thorough mixing before starting the infusion.

Do not add anything to any infusion container other than a burette when it is hanging on the infusion stand, since it makes mixing impossible.

Before adding a medicine to a hanging burette, administration must be stopped. After the addition has been made and before the administration is re-started, the contents of the burette must be carefully swirled to ensure complete mixing of the medication.

Check the appearance of the final infusion for absence of cloudiness, discolouration or particles.

Label the infusion.

Diluting a medication in a syringe for use in a pump or syringe driver

Prepare the medicine in a syringe using the appropriate method described above. Ensure labelling of syringe.

Labelling for injectable medicines/infusion containers

The person preparing the injectable medication must label the syringe immediately after preparation.

A practitioner must not be in possession of more than *one* unlabelled syringe. Labels must contain:

- the name of the patient;
- the name of the drug or drugs, if mixed;
- the dose;
- the strength;
- volume;
- diluents, if used;
- the date and the time the injectable medication was prepared;
- the signature/initial of the registered practitioner preparing the injectable medication;
- where appropriate, the date and time of expiry (Mallett & Dougherty, 2007).

The medication is now ready for administration.

Additional information that should be checked prior to administration

When administering medication, there is additional information that must be considered to reduce the risk of error and to promote the efficacy of the medication. Although some of this you may have checked in preparing the medication, once you are ready to give you should ensure that you have considered all of the following points:

The time of administration. Check against the patient's medication administration record that the medicine has not been given previously and/or is within the time band allowed. This is to ensure there is no duplication of medication and would reduce the risk of overdosing for medications that can be administered when required by the patient.

Check any instructions concerning the administration, e.g. with food or within a time window – 2 hours before food.

Check if the medication has to be delivered by a special technique.

Check if there is any additional equipment that should be used to administer the medication, e.g. a spacer being used with an inhaler.

Staff using equipment to administer medication must ensure they are familiar and are competent not only with the medication, but also with the equipment to promote the safe administration of the medicine.

Check if the medication needs to be delivered over a period of time, e.g. an intravenous injection being administered over a 2-minute period.

Is there a timing issue between drugs, e.g. multi-administration of eyedrops leaving time between installations.

Check with the summary of product characteristics if the patient requires a period of observation post-administration of the medication. This may be due to a risk of anaphylaxis or to ensure that the full effects of the medication have been achieved.

The Summary of Product Characteristics can be obtained from: www.medicines.org-uk. Pharmacists can provide additional information regarding the medication to be administered. The British National Formulary provides details of medicines information services that can be accessed for additional information.

Alternative therapies

Patients may choose to receive medicinal products that the practitioner cannot readily identify and where additional information on their use is not available within the British National Formulary.

If practitioners are administering alternative therapies, they must ensure they have the appropriate training, knowledge and competencies to administer these therapies. Practitioners may need to seek professional advice from other professionals to discuss any potential interactions or adverse effects of medication where individuals are choosing to take alternative therapies.

This issue is an ethical dilemma, since, if you do not understand the use of the drug, appropriate strength, dosage, etc., but the patient insists on using alternative therapies to manage their condition, you must respect their wishes. In this situation you should have a local policy drawn up that provides you the protection of vicarious liability from your employer and where possible you should encourage the patient to self-administer. Nonetheless, the patient's alternative medicines should all be included in the medicines administration chart and in the patient's notes.

Self-purchased medications

Individuals can self-purchase medication on the General Sales List (GSL) and Pharmacy (P) medicines. On most occasions these will be self-administered; however, if patients request to administer these preparations in the hospital or care setting, it is advisable to check with the patient's medical practitioner or prescriber to ensure it is safe to administer. An increasing number of pharmacy preparations are purchased by patients that could interact with prescription-only medicines. All such additional preparations should be written up in the patient's notes and on the patient's administration chart, since anyone prescribing for a patient, in order to act responsibly, would be required to have as much information as possible to ensure safe prescribing practice.

Post-administration of medication

Once medication has been administered, the practitioner continues to have a duty of care to the patient. The practitioner must ensure the patient or their carer has relevant information/warnings concerning the medication and its action, any side effects and how to report them. In addition, any of the following actions may be required.

- The need for follow-up blood tests/monitoring.
- The need to withhold other medication.
- The need to complete the course of medication.
- How any unused medication must be safely disposed of not only for the individual, but also for the wider community.

It is your duty as a registered practitioner to check with the prescriber and/or the summary of product characteristics to ensure you provide the appropriate information post-administration.

Record keeping

Record keeping is an essential part of the medication administration process, and this is the area that is most commonly neglected and is the subject of Nursing and Midwifery Council investigations. Practitioners must follow professional codes and employer's guidance on record keeping. The NMC guidance (2007) clearly defines the standards required. Practitioners must make clear reference in the documentation to any actions taken in relation to medication administration and that will include any advice given to patients or their carers, and any discussion with the prescriber/ lead clinician concerning the administration of the medication. If a medication is omitted, there must be a clear rationale provided in the patients' records as to the decision-making process for the omission.

Any drug errors must be reported on the employer's incident reporting documentation and policies should be in place within organizations to report such errors. These should always be within the context of a 'no blame' culture. Although registrants should make all efforts to minimize risk, the reality is mistakes will always happen. However, if a mistake occurs and the registrant fears reporting it because of managerial attitude within an organization, the consequences could be far worse. Early reporting of any error is essential to minimize the possible negative outcome.

The practitioner, if operating under a Patient Group Direction, must document the history taken to establish if a patient meets the inclusion criteria and conversely document why the patient was excluded for any reason.

Reporting errors / incidents

In the event of a medication error, the practitioner must ensure they have reported the error in accordance with organizational policies. This may include the reporting to the Medicines Healthcare Products Regulatory Agency (MHRA) of any adverse drug reaction by completion of the 'Yellow Card' that can be found in the British National Formulary or is available online from www.BNF.org.

It is essential that all adverse reactions are reported in order that licensed products may be monitored and so that, should there be a number of incidents reported on a specific product, this is identified early and appropriate action can be taken by the Medicines Healthcare Products Regulatory Agency.

Safety for staff

Patient safety is paramount when preparing and administering medication; however, there is also a need to promote safe administration for the individual staff member and their team. Infection control guidelines will promote the safe administration of the medicine for both staff and patient. Control of Substances Hazardous to Health Regulations (HSE, 2002) will inform local and national polices on the safe use of substances. Any adverse event should be reported using local policies and appropriate risk assessments should be undertaken.

The practitioner administering the medication must be aware of any necessary precautions for protection against the medication being administered. Any special precautions will be outlined in the summary of product characteristics (SPC) and it should also be clearly documented in the patient's notes that special precautions need to be taken. This may include:

- the use of protective clothing;
- the medication being prepared in a specific environment;
- reducing the risk of needle stick injury.

Following administration, it is equally important for the practitioner to be aware of polices and procedures for the safe disposal of medication. For example, this may take the form of unwanted supplies or syringes following the change within a syringe driver or pump. For specific queries that are not covered in local policies and procedures, Local Medicines Information Services (usually based in secondary care) are a useful resource where such queries should be directed.

Summary

Professional bodies, regulatory bodies, national and local organizations provide a range of policy, protocols, standards and guidelines, which outline the principles for the safe administration of medication. It is essential that you familiarize yourself with them and know their relevance. Standards as set by medicines legislation and your regulatory body must be adhered to, for these provide the broad principles under which practice must be undertaken. Local polices provide the context for which your contract of employment has been agreed. Failure to follow local policies may breach your terms and conditions and, should a case be taken against you, if local policies have not been followed, your employer may choose not to support your actions and vicarious liability for your actions may not be upheld. Best practice guidelines, however, indicate what would be considered best practice in any given situation. You may decide to provide care that goes against 'best practice'. In doing so, you should ensure that your decision was based on a clinical judgement that you can defend, that failure to act in the way you did could have posed 'risk' to the patient, and that your action could not have resulted in harm or neglect of the patient. Despite these frameworks, errors still occur with ramifications for patients, families, organizations and the individual who has administered the preparation. However, if basic principles are followed, these errors should be minimized.

Practitioners must ensure they have an up-to-date clinical and pharmaceutical knowledge base to administer medication safely. They must be competent with techniques for administration and with the equipment to be used in the administration process. They must be encouraged to acknowledge limitations in knowledge and be encouraged to undertake additional updating as required. Practitioners must be encouraged to question any aspect of the administration process if they are unclear, for they must be able to justify any actions taken with regard to the administration process.

If the practitioner adheres to the principles outlined in both national and local documents and underpins the practice of medicine administration with the principles outlined in their own profession's code of practice, the Code should be safe for the employing organization and safe for the individual practitioner. However, the most important aspect is that the administration of the medicine will be safe for the patient.

References

Alexander A, Sharma S, Mistry R. (2004) *Medicines Management Resource Pack.* Servier Laboratories Ltd.

Anderson and Anderson (1995) cited in *Manual of Clinical Nursing Procedures,* 5th edition. Editors Mallet J & Dougherty L. – The Royal Marsden Hospital. London: Blackwell Science Ltd.

Department of Health (2001a). *Medicines and Older People: Implementing Medicines Related Aspects of the NSF for Older People.* England: DH.

Department of Health (2001b). *Seeking Consent.* London: HMSO.

Department of Health (2001c). 12 *Key Points on Consent: The Law in England.* London.

Department of Health (2005). *Mental Capacity Act.* London: HMSO.

Department of Health (2006). *Health Service Circular 200/026.* London: HMSO.

Department of Health (2007a). *Medicines Matters – A Guide to Mechanisms for the Prescribing, Supply and Administration of Medicines.* London: HMSO.

Department of Health (2007b). *Safer Management of Controlled Drugs: a Guide to Good Practice in Secondary Care (England).* London.

Health and Safety Executive (2002). *COSHH: A Brief Guide to the Regulation. What You Need to Know About the Control of Substances Hazardous to Health Regulations.* London.

Mallet J & Dougherty L. (2007) *Manual of Clinical Nursing Procedures.* 5th edition – The Royal Marsden Hospital. London: Blackwell Science Ltd.

Medicines Healthcare Product Regulatory Agency (2007). *A Guide to What is a Medicinal Product.* London: MHRA.

Medicines Partnership. An Introduction to Concordance and the Medicines Partnership. http://www.medicines-partnership.org/EasySite/lib/serveDocument.asp?doc=108&pid+776.

National Patient Safety Agency (2004). *Right Patient-Right Care.* London: NPSA.

National Patient Safety Agency (2007a). Actions that can make anticoagulant therapy safer. *Patient Safety Alert 18.* London: NPSA.

National Patient Safety Agency (2007b). *Promoting Safer Measurements and*

Administration of Liquid Medicines Via Oral and Other Enteral Routes: Patient Safety Alert 19 London: NPSA.

National Patient Safety Agency (2007c). *Promoting Safer Use of Injectable Medicines: Patient Safety Alert 20.* London: NPSA.

National Patient Safety Agency (2007d). *Safety in Doses: Improving the Use of Medicines in the NHS 2007–08.* London: NPSA.

National Patient Safety Agency (2007e). *Safer Practice with Epidural Injections and Infusions:* Patient Safety Alert 21 London: NPSA.

National Prescribing Centre (2000). *Competencies for Pharmacists Working in Primary Care.* First Edition. England: NPC.

National Prescribing Centre (2007). *A Competency Framework for Shared Decision-Making with the Patients: Achieving Concordance for Taking Medicines.* NPC.

Nursing and Midwifery Council (2007a). *The Code. Standards of Conduct, Performance and Ethics for Nurses and Midwives.* London: NMC.

Nursing and Midwifery Council (2007b). *Standards of Medicine Management.* London: NMC.

Nursing and Midwifery Council (2007c). *Record Keeping.* London: NMC.

Patient UK. Patient Information leaflets. http://www.patient.co.uk/pils.asp

Royal Pharmaceutical Society of Great Britain and Merck, Sharp and Dhome (1997). *From Compliance to Concordance – Achieving Shared Goals in Medicine Taking.* London: RPSGB.

Royal Pharmaceutical Society of Great Britain and Department of Health (2006). *Safer Management of Controlled Drugs: Monitoring and Inspection Guidelines – Core Activities for Controlled Drug Monitoring and Inspection Work in Primary Care.* London: RPSGB.

Royal Pharmaceutical Society of Great Britain (2007). *Code of Ethics for Pharmacists and Pharmacy Technicians.*

Royal Pharmaceutical Society of Great Britain (2008). *British National Formulary.*

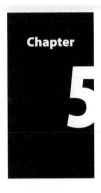

5 Adverse drug reactions and drug interactions

Tim House

This chapter aims to help you consider the problems associated with the prescribing of medicines and their management. You owe it to your patient to ensure that these issues are taken seriously. Failure to manage them can result in patient harm, loss of patient trust in your abilities, and abandonment, by the patient, of worthwhile medication.

Books on adverse drug reactions often include lists of medicines that are associated with different adverse reactions. These lists are difficult to remember and often over-simplify the facts. The first part of this chapter provides a background to adverse drug reactions. The second part looks at drug interactions where the combination of therapies can cause problems. The third part describes some information sources that can be used to manage adverse drug reactions and drug interactions. Overall the aim is to give a general background and explain how to optimize patient care.

Part 1 Adverse drug reactions

Adverse drug reactions (ADRs) are a major drain on NHS resources. In 2002, Bandolier Extra (Wiffen, 2002) stated that 7% of patients admitted to hospital are affected with ADRs. The cost to the NHS in England was estimated to be £380 million per year.

It is often difficult to decide if a patient's symptom is an ADR or a symptom of a new disease. This can lead to patients being exposed to unnecessary investigations and worry while the offending medicine is continued, and the patient continues to be exposed to its adverse effects.

What are ADRs?

Nomenclature

The World Health Organization defines adverse drug reactions as:

'A response to a drug which is noxious and unintended and which occurs at doses normally used in man for prophylaxis, diagnosis or therapy of disease, or for the modification of physiological function' (WHO, 2002).

Not all side effects of medicines are detrimental. For example, a dry mouth is a side effect of anticholinergic medicines; if an anticholinergic medicine such as orphenadrine is prescribed for Parkinson's disease, drying of the mouth will help with the excess salivation that occurs in Parkinson's disease. Metformin can cause anorexia and nausea and lead to less food consumption, which can be helpful when prescribed for an overweight type 2 diabetic.

Side effects may be so significant that they can be used as an alternative indication. For example, codeine can be used as a pain-killer, but can give the patient constipation as an unintended side effect, so codeine is also used to treat diarrhoea. Similarly, the anti-biotic erythromycin increases gastric motility and can cause diarrhoea, so is sometimes used to stimulate gastrointestinal motility in the critically ill (unlicensed use).

Type A or Type B ADRs

In 1977 Rawlins and Thompson classified ADRs into two groups, i.e. those that are pre-dictable from their pharmacology (Type A), and those that are unexpected and cannot be anticipated (Type B). Type A are 'augmented' effects and type B are 'bizarre' effects (Rawlins & Thompson, 1977).

Type A ADRs are the most common and are usually less serious. They can usually be anticipated from the medicine's pharmacology and it is often helpful to warn patients about their possible occurrence so that they will not worry about new sensations. Type A ADRs can often be managed by reducing the dose, altering the method of administra-tion or by prescribing another medicine. They are normally well documented before a drug is licensed.

Type B ADRs are normally rare, and completely unexpected, but can be potentially serious or even fatal. It is unlikely that these ADRs will have been documented before the medicine is marketed. Should a Type B ADR occur, the medicine has to be stopped as this sort of ADR is not usually dose dependent.

Examples of Type A ADRs :

- hypoglycaemia with sulphonylureas;
- unsteadiness with temazepam;
- diarrhoea with senna.

Examples of Type B ADRs include:

- anaphylaxis on administration of penicillin;
- aplastic anaemia with chloramphenicol;
- agranulocytosis with clozapine.

It is easy to think of 'typical' Type A or Type B ADRs, but some ADRs do not fall into 'typical' categories. Edwards & Aronson (2000) have extended this alphabetical clas-sification to include:

- Type C (chronic)ADRs, i.e. to include adaptive changes e.g. osteoporosis after long-term steroid use;
- Type D (delayed) ADRs, i.e. to include effects on the foetus in pregnancy, drugs in breast milk, and carcinogenesis;
- Type E (end of use), i.e. withdrawal symptoms;
- Type F (treatment failure), e.g. developing malaria while taking malaria prophylaxis.

Although easy to remember, this extended classification is not really used. In prac-tice, it is only the classification between Type A and Type B ADRs that is used, as this helps decision making with regards to treatment options.

The frequency of ADRs

For newer medicines, the Summaries of Product Characteristics (SPCs), which are the marketing authorization documents, list ADRs according to the following frequency of occurrence:

Table 5.1. Frequency of ADRs

Very common	greater than 1 in 10
Common	1 in 100 to 1 in 10
Uncommon	1 in 1000 to 1 in 100
Rare	1 in 10 000 to 1 in 1000
Very rare	less than 1 in 10 000

NB. The British National Formulary (BNF) also adopts this classification, but uses the term 'less commonly' instead of 'uncommon'.

Timelines of ADRs

ADRs most commonly appear within days or hours following the administration of the first dose of a drug. This helps diagnosis. However, in some instances, the ADR can be delayed or only occur following a cumulative dose of the drug. Such instances include the following:

- Rashes following treatment with carbamazepine, which normally appear 2 weeks to 5 months following commencement of therapy (Drugdex, 2008).
- Flucloxacillin-induced liver disease. Although the incidence of disease is higher in the first 45 days following exposure to flucloxacillin, it can present weeks after flucloxacillin has been discontinued (Russman *et al.*, 2005).
- Diethylstilboestrol was prescribed to between one and two million pregnant women to prevent pregnancy complications between the mid 1940s and the 1970s. Daughters born to these women have an increased risk of clear cell adenocarcinoma of the vagina and cervix, and their sons have an increased risk of non-cancerous epididymal cysts (Drugdex, 2008).
- The SPC for doxorubicin warns that the maximum lifetime cumulative dose must not be exceeded in order to reduce the risk of irreversible congestive heart failure.

If a symptom appears soon after a medicine has started, it is strongly indicative of an ADR. If the symptom disappears on discontinuation of the medicine, then the diagnosis becomes clearer. To confirm the diagnosis of an ADR, the medicine has to be re-introduced to see if the symptom reappears. Patients may be unwilling to participate in such an experiment, and it may be unethical as many ADRs will be worse when a medicine is re-administered.

What makes ADRs more likely?

Seniority

Elderly patients are much more likely to experience ADRs than younger patients. This is largely because the elderly are often on more medicines and suffer from more diseases than the young. Elderly patients are also physiologically less able to compensate for chemical assaults on the body, i.e. as we get older, physiological changes occur that affect the action of drugs on the body. Examples include the following:

- Protein albumin levels. Although total plasma protein levels in the blood remain relatively constant, the level of the protein albumin decreases as we get older and, as a means of compensation, the level of the protein globulin rises. This affects the activity of drugs such as warfarin and phenytoin, which bind to albumin. In the sick elderly, albumin levels tend to be even lower, and this affects the action of these two drugs to a greater extent.

- Renal function decreases with age, and so medicines such as gentamicin and digoxin are excreted less effectively. Unless gentamicin and digoxin doses are lowered, this leads to toxicity.
- Elderly patients become increasingly sensitive to certain substances including caffeine and benzodiazepines, and so may suffer adverse effects when receiving doses normally used by younger adults.

Generally, the elderly often require lower doses of many medicines compared to younger patients. As long as elderly patients are monitored, these differences should be manageable.

Neonates and children

Metabolism and excretory functions of the body are immature in neonates and children and so they are more likely, as compared to adults, to suffer ADRs. Some examples of problem areas include the following:

- Respiratory depression with morphine.
- Aspirin should not be given to children under 16 years of age because of the danger of Reye's syndrome (unless prescribed for particular indications including Kawasaki disease).
- Increased incidence of acute extrapyramidal reactions with neuroleptic drugs.
- Increased incidence of acute extrapyramidal reactions in children and young adults with metoclopramide.

Ethnic variations

The Ethnic group can affect ADRs. Examples include the following:

- Rosuvastatin blood levels in Asian patients can be double that in Caucasian or black patient groups taking the same dose of the drug. Higher doses of rosuvastatin are therefore contra-indicated in Asian patients in order to avoid ADRs.
- Increased risk of carbamazepine-induced Stevens–Johnson syndrome (a potentially fatal reaction that starts with fever and progresses to severe skin disease) among some individuals of Han Chinese, Hong Kong Chinese or Thai origin. It is now recommended that patients of these origins should be genetically screened to see if they are likely to suffer from this ADR (Drug Safety Update, 2008).

Genetic variations

Genetic variations that result in enzyme deficiencies can result in patients suffering ADRs. Examples include the following:

- Patients with glucose-6-phoshate dehydrogenase (G6PD) deficiency suffer haemolysis if given some drugs. The BNF gives a list of medicines, which included quinolone antibiotics such as ciprofloxacin.

- Some patients are deficient in the enzyme thiopurine S-methyl transferase (TPMT). Azathioprine and mercaptopurine are metabolized by this enzyme. If these drugs are given to patients with this deficiency, blood levels of the medicine build up and the patients can suffer dangerous or even fatal blood disorders.

Renal dysfunction

Renal dysfunction leads to build-up of medicines that are excreted by the kidney. If drugs such as gentamicin and digoxin are not modified to take account of this failure, they can become seriously toxic. Patients who use insulin often need lower doses of insulin in renal failure, as the kidney metabolizes insulin.

Liver disease

The liver is the organ most frequently involved in metabolizing medicines. Its malfunction can therefore result in increased potency and increased side effects of drugs. The BNF provides some basic information about the use of medicines in liver disease. This includes a vast range of medicines including all analgesics (BNF Appendix 2). Patients with liver disease are more likely to experience encephalopathy, ascites and have an increased risk of bleeding.

Gender

A greater number of ADRs are reported for females than males. Indeed, Wiffen reports that, out of 6000 hospital admissions (including 177 admissions for ADRs), 63% of the ADR-related admissions were female (Wiffen, 2002). Yellow card data show a similar ratio (Randall, 2006, p.38).

Women appear to be at greater risk of ADRs than men, possibly because of gender-related differences in pharmacokinetics, immunological and hormonal factors as well as differences in medicine use (Lee, 2006).

Examples include the following.

- Efcortesol is a brand of hydrocortisone injection (hydrocortisone sodium phosphate). In female patients paraesthesia can occur in the genital area (although it may radiate over the whole body). This is rarely reported in male patients.
- About 70% of the dystonic–dyskinetic reactions that occur in children and young people with metoclopramide are in females.

Multiple drug use

Not only do drug interactions result in opposed pharmacodynamic actions and changes in drug levels, but toxicity can occur more readily if a drug has altered or affected the patient. For example, digoxin toxicity is more pronounced if the patient is hypokalaemic. This hypokalaemia may be caused by diuretic therapy with a single agent such as furosemide, which lowers potassium levels; therefore patients on digoxin are usually prescribed a combination of furosemide and the potassium sparing diuretic amiloride (co-amilofruse).

Allergies

These are potentially very dangerous. Even a single dose of a drug that has caused an allergy can kill a patient. The issue is clouded by the large number of inaccurate allergy diagnoses. It is not unknown for patients to receive high doses of intravenous benzylpenicillin over several days and experience clear clinical benefit before it is noted they have been diagnosed in the past as having a penicillin allergy.

The situation becomes more complicated when trying to consider 'cross-sensitivities'. Cross-sensitivities occur when a patient who is allergic to one medicine is likely to be allergic to another. It is fairly easy to accept that a patient with a severe allergy to penicillin would also be allergic to amoxicillin and flucloxacillin. It is generally thought that 10% of patients with allergies to penicillin will also be allergic (have a cross-sensitivity) to cephalosporins such as cefalexin. It is not clear what proportion of patients with a penicillin allergy is unable to tolerate meropenem (Sodhi *et al.*, 2004). The immunosuppressant tacrolimus is part of the macrolide chemical family, and is contra-indicated in patients with allergy to erythromycin, clarithromycin and other macrolides.

Inappropriate administration

Examples of inappropriate administration include the following:

- Taking steroids or non-coated, non-steroidal anti-inflammatory drugs (NSAIDs) on an empty stomach can cause gastric irritation.
- Some drugs should be commenced at a low dose, and the dose increased in order to avoid an ADR. For example, lamotrigine has an increased incidence of serious skin reactions unless the patient is commenced on a low dose, and the dose is slowly increased.
- Intravenous drugs may be administered at too high a rate or concentration. If intravenous vancomycin is administered too fast, the patient is likely to suffer 'red-neck' syndrome: symptoms include erythema, flushing, or rash over the face and upper torso and sometimes hypotension, shock and possibly cardiac arrest.
- Administering intravenous potassium chloride at a rate faster than 20 mmol/h could potentially lead to cardiac arrest, although this rate has to be exceeded in some critical situations under expert supervision.

Pregnancy

Many medicines are contra-indicated in pregnancy by their Summary of Product Characteristics (SPC). However, the unborn child may be harmed to a greater extent if the mother is allowed to suffer the re-occurrence of a major disease as opposed to a medicine being prescribed. It is good practice to consider this with all female patients, as pregnancies are sometimes unplanned. If pregnancy is a possibility, expert help from a medicines information department should be considered after referral to the medicine's SPC and the pregnancy appendix of the BNF (BNF Appendix 4).

Breast-feeding

This topic is separate from pregnancy. Medicines safe in pregnancy may not be safe in breast-feeding and vice versa – look at the entry for warfarin in the pregnancy and breast-feeding appendices of the BNF. You should also note that, if a medicine is considered safe in breast-feeding, this only refers to full-term, normal weight healthy babies. Expert advice should be sought for pre-term, low birthweight or unwell babies as they may not metabolize and excrete medicines sufficiently to avoid accumulation leading to toxicity (BNF Appendix 5).

The reporting scheme for ADRs to the Commission on Human Medicines (previously the Committee on Safety of Medicines)

Pharmacovigilance is the practice that ensures the correct balance of benefit to risk of a medicine.

Thalidomide was first marketed in 1956, and was used extensively to treat nausea during pregnancy. At that time manufacturers were able to market any medicine without its safety information being assessed by a government agency.

Thalidomide was withdrawn in November 1961, following two reports of deformities. Unfortunately, due to a lack of reporting mechanisms, thousands of babies were damaged by this medicine.

In May 1964, the UK was the first country in the world to set up an adverse drug reaction database, i.e. the Yellow Card scheme. The Chairman of the Committee on Safety of Drugs, Sir Derrick Dunlop, wrote to all doctors and dentists in the UK requesting reports of 'any untoward patient conditions that might be the result of drug treatment'. He included a supply of reply-paid yellow postcards for reporting suspected reactions.

All healthcare professionals and even members of the public can report ADRs via the Yellow Card scheme. Yes this means *you*. If you suspect an ADR, you should report it unless it is a minor, already recognized ADR to an established medicine. Details about the Yellow Card scheme can be found in the BNF and at www.yellowcard.gov.uk. Yellow card reporting is covered in another chapter of this book.

Management of ADRs

Questions to ask to identify an ADR

- Have any new drugs been started?
- How soon after starting the new drug did the reaction occur?
- Could the reaction be due to the medical condition or to another disease?
- May the ADR have been precipitated by a patient factor?
- Could it have been precipitated by a drug interaction?
- Did the reaction stop when the drug was stopped?
- Did the reaction re-occur when the drug was restarted?
- Is it the drug, or an excipient that has caused the ADR? (Many patients have intolerances or allergies to excipients, e.g. lactose.)
- Is it an allergic reaction?

Which drugs are most often involved?

Research has been carried out to find out which medicines are likely to cause ADRs that result in hospital admission. One systematic review (Howard *et al.*, 2007) identified that 51% of drug-related admissions were caused by antiplatelet agents, diuretics, NSAIDs and anticoagulants. Papers included in the review were from all over the world and dated as far back as 1986. A similar study at Addenbrooke's Hospital (Bhalla *et al.*, 2003) found that cardiovascular and central nervous system drugs (including alcohol abuse) represented 67% of ADR related admissions. NSAIDs represented 12.5% of admissions. This is in line with Howard *et al.*'s (2007) finding of 11% NSAID associated admissions.

What action should be taken to manage the ADR?

- Check that the medicine is being taken correctly. Some medicines (e.g. ibuprofen) will upset the stomach; this ADR can be alleviated if the patient takes the medicine with food. Dexamethasone is used frequently in oncology for a variety of indications; but it can cause restlessness, which can greatly interfere with the sleep of the patient and therefore will keep their partner awake as well. This is less likely to occur if the last dose is taken no later than 6 pm.
- Anticipate and treat, e.g. prescribe anti-emetics for a patient before commencing chemotherapy. If an NSAID is prescribed for a patient at risk of gastro-intestinal bleeding, co-prescribe omeprazole or misoprostol.
- Decide if it is a type A or B ADR. If it is type B, then discontinue immediately, and select a different therapy. This may need to be from a different class of medicines. If it is a Type A ADR, then dose reduction may solve the problem.
- Find out if it is reversible. If not, discontinue and seek advice about treatment of the ADR.
- Find out if tolerance will develop. Patients started on nitrates for cardiac disease very often develop headaches caused by the vasodilation. Tolerance develops to this ADR after a week or so. If this is explained to the patient, they are likely to adhere to this life-saving therapy.
- Consider whether the benefit of the treatment is great enough to endure the ADR. For example, oral acetazolamide is often given to patients who have dangerously raised intraocular pressure. Acetazolamide causes pins and needles, nausea and depression, but tolerating a few days of this unpleasant medicine can prevent patients from losing their eyesight. Similarly, many chemotherapies cause a patient to lose their hair, but they can prolong their life.

Some adverse drug reaction groups

We could provide lists of medicines that are associated with a large number of individual ADRs but these are arbitrary and difficult to remember. It may be helpful to examine some groups of ADRs so that they can be anticipated. Sometimes the expression used is 'side effect', as the effect may or may not be an adverse reaction, depending on the patient's symptoms.

Rashes

Rashes are fairly simple – any drug can cause any type of skin rash or eruption. Indeed, some authors suggest a shortlist of medicines that do not cause skin problems. These include digoxin, inorganic compounds such as ferrous sulphate and potassium chloride, and vitamins (Arndt & Jick, 1976).

Rashes are one of the most common adverse effects related to medicines. About one in five Yellow Card Reports are for rashes. Most of these ADRs will occur within 1 week of therapy initiation but some, including carbamazepine rashes (see above) occur typically 1 month following the initiation of therapy.

Rashes as part of hypersensitivity reactions to penicillins can occur several weeks after the discontinuation of therapy and reactions to gold can occur even later. Another example of a delayed reaction is the beta-blocker practolol (now withdrawn), which could sometimes produce a rash more than a year after therapy commenced.

Other factors can influence the incidence of skin rashes. For example, 95% of patients with infectious mononucleosis and treated with ampicillin develop a rash (Pullen *et al.*, 1967). Another example is that HIV-positive patients are ten times more likely to experience skin reactions when prescribed co-trimoxazole than HIV-negative patients (De Raeve, 1988).

Not all rashes are trivial, i.e. angio-oedema, erythroderma, Stevens–Johnson syndrome and toxic epidermal necrolysis can be severe and potentially life-threatening.

Antimuscarinic (anticholinergic) side effects

Antimuscarinic (anticholinergic) side effects are predictable from the pharmacology of the autonomic nervous system and so they are classic Type A ADRs. Side effects include:

- slowing of gut motility leading to constipation;
- restricting of the bladder opening leading to urinary retention;
- dilated pupils resulting in blurred vision (the dilation can be a danger if patients are at risk of angle-closure glaucoma);
- dryness of the mouth with difficulty in swallowing and talking;
- thirst;
- transient bradycardia, followed by tachycardia with the possibility of palpitations and arrhythmias.

Medicines likely to cause these ADRs are anticholinergic medicines such as oxybutynin, tricyclic antidepressants, antihistamines and phenothiazines (e.g. prochlorperazine).

These medicines should be avoided in patients with gastro-intestinal obstruction and myasthenia gravis. They should also be used with caution in patients with various co-morbidities including cardiac disease and prostatic hypertrophy.

Cholinergic side effects

Not many medicines have cholinergic side effects. An example is pilocarpine, which is a licensed oral medication for the treatment of dry mouth. These side effects are easy to predict as they are the opposite of anticholinergic side effects. They include:

- diarrhoea;
- urinary frequency;

- excess sweating;
- drooling;
- clammy skin.

Serotonin syndrome and neuroleptic malignant syndrome

Serotonin syndrome and neuroleptic malignant syndrome are rare but potentially life-threatening adverse reactions. Symptoms of serotonin syndrome can include confusion, disorientation, abnormal movements, exaggerated reflexes, fever, sweating, diarrhoea and hypotension or hypertension. If three or more of these symptoms are present without any other explanation for their cause, then serotonin syndrome is diagnosed. This condition can be fatal, although it is usually mild and will resolve when the offending medicine (or combination of medicines) has been stopped. Serotonin syndrome occurs most commonly if more than one drug that affects the serotonin system is taken, e.g. if adding fluoxetine to amitriptyline, or even replacing one medicine that affects the serotonin system with another. There have also been case reports of serotonin syndrome when patients have been taking only one agent, e.g. venlafaxine.

Neuroleptic malignant syndrome is rare but dangerous. Symptoms include fever (with high temperature), extreme rigidity, autonomic instability, and changes in mental status. This syndrome normally occurs when patients are taking neuroleptic agents, or medicines that affect dopamine neurotransmission. After the offending drugs have been stopped, treatment with dantrolene or bromocriptine is normally given.

Extrapyramidal symptoms

Antipsychotic drugs commonly cause extrapyramidal symptoms, which are movement disorders. The BNF describes these symptoms and advises that they occur most frequently with piperazine phenothiazines (fluphenazine, perphenazine, prochlorperazine and trifluoperazine), the butyrophenones (benperidol and haloperidol) and depot preparations of these medicines. Some of the symptoms are not reversible (BNF 4.2.1).

Opioid side effects

Opioids have a range of adverse effects that are predictable and should be anticipated. Drowsiness, confusion and nausea are likely to occur when starting opioids. The patient will become tolerant to these adverse effects, but they will reappear at each dose increase. Opioids also cause constipation, but patients will not develop tolerance to this side effect, and constipation will worsen after each dose increase. If prescribing potent opioids, laxatives should routinely be prescribed, and laxative doses reviewed, with the expectation of increasing the dose each time the opioid dose is increased. Opioids can also cause respiratory depression, but usually this will only occur if the dose is too high.

Beta-blockers

By virtue of their pharmacology, beta-blockers slow body systems and reduce the work of the heart. This means, in practice, that patients will often feel worse when starting these medications and complain of tiredness, lack of interest and cold extremities.

Asthmatic patients, and patients with obstructive pulmonary disease, experience a worsening of their condition if given these medicines. Therefore, beta-blockers should not be prescribed for these patients.

It is important to remember that eye drops containing beta-blockers (e.g. timolol) may cause these side effects as absorption can be significant. Up to May 1990, the CSM had received 66 reports of bronchospasm, suspected following the use of beta-blocker eye drops, three of which were fatal (Anon, 1990).

Blood dyscrasias

Agranulocytosis is a rare but potentially fatal decrease in white cell count that will seriously reduce a patient's ability to fight infection. This can occur with medicines such as clozapine, gold salts, azathioprine or carbimazole (a Type B ADR). Patients taking these medicines should be advised to watch for signs of infection such as fever or sore throat and to have a blood test if these symptoms occur.

Many chemotherapy agents interfere with blood cell generation because they work by interfering with cell replication (both in malignant cells and healthy cells) involved in the production of blood cells. The patient will have a dangerously low white cell count and be susceptible to infection whilst receiving these therapies. Anti-microbial therapy should be co-prescribed with these agents, as the patient will have difficulty overcoming an infection because of their reduced white cell count.

Non-steroidal anti-inflammatory drugs (NSAIDs)

Bleeds, kidney damage and hypertension are common side effects of NSAIDs. The elderly are particularly prone to ADRs caused by these medicines. Gastro-intestinal bleeds often occur without prior stomach pain, probably because the analgesic effect of the NSAID relieves the pain that would have given the patient advance warning of danger.

Additionally, in some individuals, asthma symptoms can be worsened; even topical NSAID preparations (e.g. felbinac, piroxicam gels) have been reported to cause bronchospasm.

Conclusion to ADR section

If a medicine has potential for benefit, it probably has potential for harm. The prescriber and patient should discuss the benefits and potential harmful effects of each medicine. Without careful management, potentially beneficial treatments may be abandoned or patients may be harmed.

Part 2 Drug interactions

Drug interactions occur when two or more drugs interact in such a way that the effectiveness or toxicity of one or more of the drugs is altered. Dietary supplements, herbal medicines, alcohol, cigarettes and food are agents that can cause interactions.

The aim of this part of the chapter is to give a broad background to drug interactions so that you will understand them and be aware of the medicines that are commonly involved in clinically important interactions.

Broadly speaking drug interactions fall within two groups: pharmacodynamic and pharmakokinetic.

Pharmacodynamic

These interactions occur when a medicine modifies the effect of another medicine but without altering the blood level of that medicine.

Examples include:

- Co-administration of a beta-blocker (e.g. propranolol or atenolol) with a beta-agonist (e.g. salbutamol either oral or inhaled). The beta-blocker blocks the beta-receptors in the lower respiratory tract potentially giving rise to bronchospasm and limiting the effectiveness of the beta-agonist.
- The combination of ACE inhibitors (e g. enalapril or lisinopril) and potassium sparing diuretics (e.g. amiloride in co-amilofruse). As both agents increase potassium levels, this can lead to dangerous or even fatal hyperkalaemia, particularly in patients with poor renal function.
- Serotonin syndrome already discussed in the ADR section.
- Drowsiness caused by alcohol exacerbates the drowsiness caused by sedating medicines.

Pharmacokinetic

These interactions involve one drug altering another drug's blood level, during absorption, distribution, metabolism or excretion.

Interaction at site of absorption

- Mixing intravenous drugs prior to administration may cause formation of a precipitate, which results in loss of activity and the danger of clots forming in the vein. Therefore, it is important that injections are not mixed, even in the same IV line, unless compatibility has been proven.
- Interaction at the site of absorption can also occur with oral medicines, e.g. heavy metal ions such as calcium and magnesium will precipitate with antibiotics such as tetracyclines or quinolones (e.g. ciprofloxacin and norfloxacin). The antibiotic is then not absorbed and treatment failure can occur. The quinolone antibiotic norfloxacin, and calcium supplements, are both given twice daily. If calcium is taken at the same time, the absorption of norfloxacin can be reduced by as much as 60% (Stockley, 2008). Patients need to avoid indigestion remedies and milk products around the times of taking these medications to optimize absorption.
- Colestyramine will absorb many drugs, resulting in drugs not being absorbed by the body. Medicines particularly affected include digoxin, tetracyclines and warfarin (Stockley, 2008).
- Problems can occur if a drug reduces the acidity of the stomach. For example, ketoconazole absorption is reduced by ranitidine or indigestion remedies that change the stomach from an acid to alkaline environment.

Distribution interactions

Many medicines are bound to the albumin component of plasma proteins. It is possible to quantify the proportion of the medicine actually bound to the plasma protein, e.g.

phenytoin is 90%–93% bound to protein and the figures for lisinopril, penicillin V and warfarin are 3%–10%, 80% and 97%–99.5%, respectively (Dollery, 1999). It is important to understand that the medicine actually bound to the protein is out of reach, i.e. it cannot provide any therapeutic benefit or cause any ADR. When blood levels are measured, the total level of the medicine is measured including both the plasma bound and the free (unbound) medicine.

When medicines are highly protein bound (at least 90%), significant danger can occur. If a patient is established on a highly protein-bound medicine, and is then started on another medicine that is also protein bound, the new medicine may displace some or all the established medicine from the protein. This means the free level of the established medicine increases greatly, so it becomes more active and potentially toxic. What then happens is that the excess free established medicine is metabolized, and the original ratio of bound to unbound is re-established. Therefore, in practice this interaction rarely causes harm.

One potentially toxic example is the prescribing of sodium valproate for patients already established on the highly protein-bound phenytoin. Here the sodium valproate displaces the phenytoin and the level of free phenytoin becomes very high. The maximum rate at which the body can metabolize phenytoin may be exceeded, and so it will take days to return to the previous bound to unbound ratio. Meanwhile, high free phenytoin levels can cause toxicity even though the measurement of blood levels (bound plus unbound) may suggest sub-therapeutic blood levels (this interaction is further complicated as phenytoin enhances the metabolism of sodium valproate, and sodium valproate inhibits the metabolism of phenytoin).

Metabolism interactions

Many medicines are metabolized by enzymes and removed via breath, urine or faeces. The cytochrome P450 enzyme family is particularly important. Each member of this enzyme family has its own range of medicines that it can metabolize. Additionally, some medicines induce or inhibit these individual enzymes, which lead to drug interactions.

It is not necessary to get too involved in the biochemistry, but you should know that these enzymes have names like 2B6, 2C9, 2C19, 2D6, 2E1 and 3A4. The most important enzymes are the 3A4 group.

If you know which specific enzymes metabolize a particular medicine, and you know which medicines induce or inhibit that enzyme, then you can understand and predict drug interactions.

For example, simvastatin is a substrate of 3A4; its metabolism will be increased by rifampicin (an inducer of 3A4) and reduced by clarithromycin (an inhibitor of 3A4). This means that simvastatin will become less effective if rifampicin is prescribed, but can become toxic if clarithromycin is prescribed. Meanwhile, ethanol will not affect simvastatin as ethanol affects only 2C9 and 2E1 enzymes.

Carbamazepine stimulates the enzymes that metabolize itself. This is why the dose of carbamazepine is initiated at a low dose, and then increased slowly. Not only does the metabolism of carbamazepine increase but, by inducing the enzymes, other drugs including warfarin, diltiazem and ciclosporin will also be metabolized more rapidly, reducing their effect. Carbamazepine is metabolized by at least five of these enzymes, but importantly by 3A4. Warfarin, diltiazem and ciclosporin are metabolized by 3A4, therefore they will be metabolized faster and their blood levels will fall. On the other hand, diltiazem inhibits the 3A4 enzyme. So, in a patient stabilized on carbamazepine, starting diltiazem will result in 3A4 inhibition, which results in less metabolism of carbamazepine; carbamazepine blood levels will increase and the patient may show signs of toxicity, typically double vision.

Although cytochrome P450 enzymes are thought of as liver enzymes, they can also be found in other locations including the mucosa of the gastro-intestinal tract. Constituents of grapefruit juice inhibit 3A4 just the same as clarithromycin or diltiazem. There are reports of increases of about 70% in blood levels when grapefruit juice has been taken with oral ciclosporin. On the other hand, a study of intravenous ciclosporin and oral grapefruit juice showed no elevation of ciclosporin levels, which implies it is the gut wall cytochrome enzymes that are being affected (Stockley, 2008).

The CHM has advised that grapefruit juice should be totally avoided in patients on simvastatin. Patients taking atorvastatin should avoid large quantities of grapefruit juice, but fluvastatin, pravastatin and rosuvastatin can be taken with grapefruit juice as they are not metabolized substantially by CYP3A4.

There are also issues about grapefruit juice and calcium channel blockers. The bio-availability of calcium channel blockers is increased by grapefruit juice and some manu-facturers instruct to avoid taking grapefruit juice with their calcium channel blocker. Apart from felodipine and nisoldipine, Stockley concludes that the interaction is likely to be of little clinical significance (Stockley, 2008).

The CSM advised that cranberry juice should be avoided in patients taking warfarin as it can raise the INR. One patient died and it was suspected that a combination of cranberry juice and warfarin was the cause (Anon, 2003).

Enhancement of liver enzymes requires new enzyme to be produced and so a full effect will not be seen for between 1 and 3 weeks. Enzyme inhibitors will show their effect within 24 hours.

Drugs with long half-lives can also cause problems. Fluoxetine and its active metab-olite have a half-life of 5–15 days. Amiodarone has a half-life of about 52 days. So, these drugs can produce interactions even if they were stopped weeks previously.

Persistent excessive alcohol consumption leads to enhanced liver enzymes activity, so regular high alcohol consumption can result in lower levels of medicines such as warfarin and phenytoin.

Alcohol abuse can be treated with disulfiram, which interacts with alcohol. The body converts alcohol to acetaldehyde and then the enzyme acetaldehyde dehydrogen-ase metabolizes the acetaldehyde. Disulfiram inhibits this enzyme and the unpleasant chemical acetaldehyde builds up in the blood, leading to flushing, breathlessness, tachy-cardia, giddiness, hypotension, nausea and vomiting. This discourages further alcohol consumption.

There is debate as to whether this disulfiram reaction also occurs with metronida-zole. There is little evidence to support the avoidance of alcohol while taking metroni-dazole, although the SPC for Flagyl advises against alcohol during therapy and for 48 hours after completion of the course. As metronidazole is normally only given for short courses, it is prudent to follow this advice. The only problem is that, if you tell a patient they should not take alcohol and metronidazole together, they may choose to take just the alcohol.

Table 5.2. Some important interacting agents involving P450 enzymes

Enzyme inducers	Enzyme inhibitors	Enzyme substrates
Barbiturates	Amiodarone	Amiodarone
Carbamazepine	Cimetidine, ciprofloxacin	Ciclosporin
Phenytoin	Clarithromycin, diltiazem	Nifedipine
Rifampicin	Erythromycin, fluconazole	Phenytoin
St John's wort	Fluoxetine, itraconazole	Simvastatin
	Ketoconazole, metronidazole	Theophylline
	Verapamil	Warfarin

Cigarette smoking stimulates liver enzymes that metabolize theophylline, so smokers need higher doses of theophylline. On smoking cessation, theophylline doses need to be decreased by one-quarter or one-third after 1 week's abstinence, and reduced further over the next months.

Dietary supplements often include vitamins and minerals that may interact like normal medicines. Patients often believe herbal preparations to be safe, but they can interact in similar ways to mainstream medicines. St John's wort is a significant enzyme inducer of cytochrome P450 3A4. Other herbs that can interact with medicines include feverfew, garlic, ginkgo, ginseng and dandelion. With all herbs, there is considerable difference in potency between manufacturers and even batches from the same manufacturer.

You should remember the following examples of enzyme inducers, enzyme inhibitors and enzyme substrates in Table 5.2, so that you can anticipate drug interactions. This is not an exhaustive list, but these are the medicines you are more likely to come across in practice and should automatically put you into an interaction frame of mind. If you deal with transplant or HIV patients, then their medicines should also be added to this list, as they commonly interact via CYP450 enzymes.

NB. Enzyme inducers and inhibitors are usually substrates as well.

Excretion interactions

Some drugs reduce renal blood flow, and so reduce the renal elimination of drugs. For example, NSAIDs may reduce renal blood flow, which can lead to the reduction in excretion of drugs such as methotrexate and lithium. This leads to elevated blood levels and potential toxicity. Patients with rheumatoid arthritis often receive NSAIDs and low-dose weekly methotrexate. Rheumatologists often prescribe this combination, but monitor the patient carefully.

Probenecid competes with penicillin for excretion via the kidney, which slows the elimination of the penicillin. In the early days of penicillin manufacture the production was very limited and this interaction was actively exploited to maximize the number of patients that could be treated. Readers of Graham Greene's *The Third Man* will know that, in 1949 Vienna, benzylpenicillin was only available to military hospitals and Harry Lime was involved in the black market of benzylpenicillin injections at a price of £70 per vial. We still exploit this interaction among syphilis patients so that a long-acting penicillin injection can be given just once a day when co-prescribed with probenecid.

Identifying potentially harmful drug interactions and how to manage them in clinical practice

Medicines that require particular care where there are potential drug interactions

- Drugs with narrow therapeutic margins, e.g. warfarin, digoxin, antiepileptics, theophylline, ciclosporin and tacrolimus.
- Drugs that require careful dosage control, e.g. antihypertensives and antidiabetic drugs.

Medicines that are likely to be implicated in drug interactions

Table 5.3. Some medicines commonly involved in drug interactions

Warfarin	Rifampicin
Salts of metals e.g. Ca, Mg, Zn, Fe	Antiepileptics
Erythromycin and clarithromycin	Theophylline and aminophylline
Amiodarone	Ciclosporin, tacrolimus, sirolimus
Diltiazem, verapamil	Ciprofloxacin
Omeprazole	Antifungals

Ways of managing drug interactions include:

- Changing administration times, e.g. calcium supplements with ciprofloxacin. The SPC for ciproxin advises that calcium should not be administered within 4 hours of ciprofloxacin.
- Changing the dose in anticipation, e.g. the BNF advises halving the dose of digoxin if adding amiodarone.
- TDM (therapeutic drug monitoring), measuring the blood levels of drugs when they interact, e.g. monitoring the blood level of theophylline when ciprofloxacin is added.
- Monitoring for side effects, e.g. watching for bruising when adding drugs that interact with the patient's warfarin.
- Temporarily stopping one therapy, e.g. the SPC for Zocor (simvastatin) states that simvastatin should be stopped while a patient is taking erythromycin.
- Changing the drug to a different drug in the same class, which does not interact, or interacts to a lesser extent, e.g. changing fluoxetine to citalopram.
- Remembering that, when an interacting medicine is stopped, the interaction will be reversed.

Part 3 Information sources

The British National Formulary (BNF)

This convenient book is readily available and updated every 6 months. ADRs are listed in approximate order of frequency arranged broadly by body systems. Occasionally, a rare side effect might be listed first if it is considered to be particularly serious. For drug interactions, Appendix 1 is a handy, easily accessible source. It is abbreviated to be practical; so warfarin is under coumarins, etc. You will note that some interactions are blobbed (have a ● at the side) which means the interaction is 'potentially hazardous' and combined administration should be avoided or used only with caution and appropriate monitoring. This can be accessed over the internet at www.bnf.org.

Summary of product characteristics (SPCs)

A medicine's SPC is its official licence document. This lists the ADRs that a medicine is associated with, referring to them as 'undesirable effects'. There are also sections on the suitability of the medicine in pregnancy and lactation, and also a section on interactions with other medicinal products. This is best accessed over the internet at www.medicines.org.uk. Alternatively, a printed copy (the *Medicines Compendium* – published annually) can be obtained by ordering from the website. There are disadvantages in having a printed copy, not only is it heavy, but it will be out of date before you receive it.

It should be remembered that not all SPCs are available this way. SPCs for generic medicines are frequently not available but the SPC of original patented medicine may still be available, and the information will effectively be valid.

Adverse Drug Reactions

This is a well-referenced and practical book that helps in the understanding, identification and management of ADRs. *Adverse Drug Reactions*, 2nd edn (2006), Lee A (Ed), London: Pharmaceutical Press.

Yellow Card data

Data obtained from the Yellow Card reports are now available over the internet at www.yellowcard.gov.uk. Key limiting factors to the database's usefulness for quantifying side effects are the following:

- Unknown rate of use of drug.
- Unknown degree of under-reporting; it is often suggested that only 1 in 20 reportable ADRs are reported. Some patient groups may be more likely to report certain adverse effects than others.
- There is no indication of seriousness or severity.
- Doses, routes and indications are not recorded. This is particularly difficult with medicines such as aspirin where the most common dose now is 75 mg daily for its antiplatelet effect, when in the past it had been taken in doses of up to 4 g daily

for its analgesic effect. Similarly, methotrexate patients can receive between 7.5 mg weekly and massive IV doses as high as 25 g.

- These are only *suspected* ADRs and not proven.

Stockley's Drug Interactions

This is the most respected text on drug interactions describing mechanisms of interactions and advising on their management. *Stockley's Drug Interactions,* 8th edn (2008), Baxter K (Ed.), London: Pharmaceutical Press.

Cytochrome P450 databases

There are various lists of drugs that are affected by or affect P450 enzymes. These can be used to anticipate drug interactions. One example is http://medicine.iupui.edu/flockhart/table.htm.

Medicines information departments

Most hospitals have medicines information departments that are pharmacy run to provide an enquiry answering service of matters relating to medicines. They have more specialized reference sources and expertise in advising on such issues as ADRs, drug interactions and the use of medicines in pregnancy and breast-feeding.

Medical information departments

Manufacturers are under an obligation to provide an information service for their medicines and are also under an obligation to follow up and report any suspected adverse reaction to their medicine. It should be remembered that they can only deal with enquiries about their own medicines.

Conclusion

It is not possible in one chapter to include all the information that is needed to manage ADRs and drug interactions. The chapter has aimed to give a basic understanding of the more common issues and to indicate where further information can be found.

References

Anon (1990). Bronchospasm associated with cardioselective and topical beta-blockers. *Committee on Safety of Medicines. Current Problems No. 28.*

Anon (2003). Possible interaction between warfarin and cranberry juice. *Current Problems in Pharmacovigilance,* **29**, 8.

Arndt JK, Jick H. (1976). Rates of cutaneous reactions to drugs. A report of the Boston Drug Surveillance Programme. *Journal of the American Medical Association,* **235**, 918–23.

Bhalla N, Duggan C, Dhillon S. (2003). The incidence and nature of drug-related admissions to hospital. *Pharmaceutical Journal,* **270**, 583–6.

BNF. (British National Formulary) March 2009 57th edn, London: BMJ Group/RPS Publishing. Available at www.bnf.org.

De Raeve L, Song M, van Maldergem L. (1988). Adverse cutaneous reaction in AIDS. *British Journal of Dermatology,* **119**, 521–3.

Dollery C. (ed.) (1999). *Therapeutic Drugs.* 2nd edn. Edinburgh: Churchill Livingstone.

Drug Safety Update (2008). Carbamazepine: genetic testing recommended in some Asian populations. *Drug Safety Update*, **1**, 5.

Drugdex (2008). Klasco RK. (ed.) Drugdex System. *Thomson Healthcare, Greenwood Village, Colorado* (Vol. **136**, expires June 2008).

Edwards JR, Aronson JK. (2000). Adverse drug reactions: definitions, diagnosis and management. *Lancet*, **356**, 1255–9.

Howard RL, Avery AJ, Slavenburg S, Royal S, Pipe G, Lucassen P, Primohamed M, *et al.* (2007). Which drugs cause preventable admissions to hospital? A systematic review. *British Journal of Clinical Pharmacology*, **63** (2), 136–47.

Lee A. (ed.) (2006). *Adverse Drug Reactions*. 2nd edn. London: Pharmaceutical Press.

Pullen H, Wright N, Murdoch JMcC. (1967). Hypersensitivity reactions to antibacterial drugs in infectious mononucleosis. *Lancet*, ***ii***, 1176–8.

Randall C. (ed.) (2006). Adverse drug reactions, an open learning programme for pharmacists. 4th edn. *Centre for Pharmacy Postgraduate Education*. University of Manchester.

Rawlins MD, Thompson JW. (1977). Pathogenesis of adverse drug reactions. In Davies DM. (ed.) *Textbooks of Adverse Drug Reactions*. Oxford: Oxford University Press.

Russman S, Haye JA, Jick SS, *et al.* (2005). Risk of cholestatic liver disease associated with flucloxacillin and flucloxacillin prescribing habits in the UK: cohort study using data from the UK General Practice Research Database. *British Journal of Clinical Pharmacology*, **60**, 76–82.

Stockley IH. (2008). *Stockley's Drug Interactions*, Baxter, K., ed. 8th edn. London: Pharmaceutical Press.

Sodhi M, Astell S, *et al.* (2004). Is it safe to use carbapenems in patients with a history of allergy to penicillin? *Journal of Antimicrobial Chemotherapy*, **54**, 1155–7.

WHO (2002). The importance of pharmacovigilance p 40. Accessed at http://www.who.int/medicinedocs/collect/edmweb/pdf/s4893e/s4893e.pdf July 2008.

Wiffen P, Gill M, *et al.* (2002) Adverse drug reactions in hospital patients. A systematic review of the prospective and retrospective studies. Bandolier Extra June 2002. Accessed at http://www.medicine.ox.ac.uk/bandolier/Extraforbando/ADRPM.pdf July 2008.

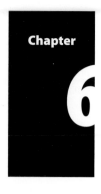

Interface of care and communication

Alison Blenkinsopp, Gill Dorer, Martin Duerden, Rebecca Jester

Objectives

Identify the types of medication problems that arise at transition points in primary healthcare.

Explore the reasons why these problems occur.

Discuss possible methods of improving patient safety.

Summary

Interfaces and transitions relating to medicines use occur across healthcare settings and between healthcare professionals. This chapter focuses on primary care where the majority of medicines are prescribed and used. Medicines related problems (MRPs) have effects ranging from inconvenience, through impaired quality of life, to serious harm. There is increasing evidence that many MRPs are caused by communication failures and that future solutions need to include tackling the human causes of inadequate communication. Four medicines (anticoagulants, diuretics, non-steroidal anti-inflammatories and antiplatelet medicines) are responsible for half of the medicines related hospital admissions and many of these episodes could be prevented with improved surveillance and interventions in primary care. Possible solutions are discussed including proactive monitoring in partnership with patients (including clinicians not making assumptions that someone else has ensured safety), the use of medicines review, and methods of strengthening patients' and carers' knowledge. All healthcare professionals should be vigilant and not assume that the correct prescription, supply, appropriateness and safety of medication has been checked already. Clinicians need to give adequate information to patients and check the patient's or carer's knowledge at each stage. Patients should be regarded as experts in their own conditions and be encouraged to flag up any concerns.

In this chapter we first consider the relevant *background* of causes and consequences of problems with medicines at interfaces in care before going into greater detail about the *four medicines* that are responsible for most hospital admissions. We then go on to discuss *possible solutions* before drawing our *conclusions*.

Background

Medicines related problems (MRPs – including, for example, over- or under-dosing and adverse effects) are common throughout the healthcare system and occur at all points in the therapeutic chain from prescribing, through dispensing to the use of medicines by patients. A recent review noted that *many adverse drug events result from problems with communication relating to management of drugs during the transition between care settings* (Spinewine, 2008). The effects of MRPs and attempts to solve them include:

inconvenience and confusion to the patient;

patient losing confidence in the clinician;

waste of healthcare professional's time;

sub-optimal use of medicines;

impaired quality of life;

potential or actual harm;

potential for litigation.

One potential consequence is admission to hospital resulting from, or related to, medication. However, hospital admissions represent the tip of a large iceberg of impaired health resulting from medication. Although adverse drug reaction data are frequently (but incompletely) collated, data on patients' experience of symptoms related to medicines are sparse with the exception of a large study involving over 600 patients from four primary care medical practices in the USA. A quarter of these patients identified a total of 286 medication-related symptoms but had discussed only two-thirds of these with their doctor. The doctors had changed therapy in response to three-quarters of the symptoms reported by patients and there were differences in individual doctors' propensity to change medication in response to patients' reports. The researchers concluded that '*Primary care physicians may be able to reduce the duration and/or the severity of many ADEs by eliciting and addressing patients' medication symptoms*' (Weingart *et al.*, 2005).

Queries from community pharmacists to prescribers relating to prescriptions are commonplace in primary care and there are some studies of the incidence and nature of pharmacists' interventions. One UK study found that pharmacists in nine community pharmacies over a 1-month period intervened in 0.6% of the prescription items dispensed (Chen *et al.*, 2005). Prescriptions containing incomplete or incorrect information accounted for two-thirds of the problems. A US study of 'pharmacy callbacks' where the community pharmacist telephones the primary care medical practice to clarify a prescription prior to dispensing involved recording of pharmacist queries by 22 practices over a 2-week period (Hansen *et al.*, 2006). Ambiguities in dosage, instructions, type of medicine, amount and illegibility were frequently recorded. Queries were resolved the same day in around two-thirds of cases but nevertheless led to delays in dispensing. Interestingly, the researchers found higher numbers of queries in training practices with trainee family doctors, an aspect which has not yet been explored in the UK literature.

Preventable medication-related hospital admissions have been the subject of many studies over the years. A recent systematic review found that over half of preventable drug-related admissions involved either antiplatelets (16%), diuretics (16%), non-steroidal anti-inflammatory drugs (11%) or anticoagulants (8%) (Howard *et al.*, 2007). Of those admissions that were judged to be preventable, one-third were due to prescribing problems, a further third to adherence problems and one in five to monitoring problems. The same research team conducted a qualitative study involving patients, carers, primary care physicians, community pharmacists and practice nurses to understand the reasons that problems had occurred and to consider possible improvement strategies (Howard *et al.*, 2008). They concluded that '*the main causes of these problems are communication failures (between patients and healthcare professionals and different groups of healthcare professionals) and knowledge gaps (about drugs and patients' medical and medication histories)'.*

There was reluctance among the community pharmacists in the study to challenge even a patient's prescription that they suspected might be harmful. The reason that pharmacists gave for this was that they had insufficient information about patients' medical history and about why a specific medicine had been selected. Primary care physicians in the study reported problems accessing and cross-referencing information in complex electronic patient records (the report of the study mentions blood tests being separate from diagnosis, for example) and failures in updating patient records after a home visit meant the information was incomplete. Interaction alerts on both Primary care physicians' and pharmacy computer systems were also identified as a problem. This may be at least partly because clinicians 'tune' out when receiving many so-called 'nag screens' from their computer software. There is also evidence from a US study that '*Pharmacists override a substantial proportion of drug-interaction alerts of minor or moderate potential severity by ignoring them or by programming the system to only flag drug interactions of potentially high severity*' (Indermitte *et al.*, 2007). The UK researchers recommended training to improve communication between prescribers and pharmacists so that pharmacists would find it less difficult to challenge potential problems in prescriptions. An obvious solution would be to have a unified record between pharmacy and general practice, such as an electronic patient record accessible to both. Alternatively, a patient-held electronic record could be used.

Further evidence of the contribution of inadequate communication to medicines related hospital admissions comes from a study of over 100 patients aged 75 or over and who had been readmitted to hospital as an emergency within 28 days of previous discharge (Witherington *et al.*, 2008). Documentation of changes in medication was incomplete on two-thirds of all discharge documents. Readmission was considered to be related to medication in 40% of cases and to be preventable for almost two-thirds of these. The researchers found preventable discharge communication gaps, including monitoring information, for half of these patients. The authors concluded that '*incomplete documentation at discharge was common, particularly for medication management. It is likely that communication gaps contributed to many of the preventable adverse events and readmissions*'. This has become the focus of recent strategies based around medicines reconciliation, now the subject of guidance from the National Institute for Health and Clinical Excellence (NICE) and National Patient Safety Agency (NPSA). Medicines Reconciliation has been defined as '*the process of identifying the most accurate list of a patient's current medicines – including the name, dosage, frequency, and route – and comparing them to the current list you are working from, recognizing any discrepancies, and documenting any changes, thus resulting in a complete list of medications, accurately communicated*' (Institute of Healthcare Improvement). A common example of things going wrong when a patient is discharged from hospital is the patient's antihypertensive medication not being included in the 'to take out' medicines because, while in hospital, the patient's blood pressure dropped perhaps because of intra-operative blood loss and the use of opioid analgesics. In primary care it may be assumed that the antihypertensive has been stopped deliberately and permanently. The patient's blood pressure then gradually increases after going home and this may not be spotted.

In the next section of this chapter we take the four medicines identified as responsible for the majority of hospital admissions and attempt to unpick the evidence for what and how things go wrong.

Medication safety exemplars

The case of warfarin

Increasing numbers of patients are being prescribed warfarin and this trend is likely to accelerate, given recent trials evidence that warfarin is preferable to aspirin in older people with atrial fibrillation; for many, the increased risks related to bleeding are outweighed by benefits in stroke reduction. Although more anticoagulation monitoring services are now provided in primary care, and some patients now self-monitor, many patients still have to go to hospital for INR monitoring. Transitions between the interfaces between the hospital clinic, the GP practice and the dispensing pharmacy and the patient are not currently robust enough. The risks that the NPSA identified as contributing to serious ADEs involving anticoagulants are shown in Box 6.1 and led to an alert being issued in 2007 (Baglin *et al.*, 2006).

Box 6.1. Risks identified from the NPSA anticoagulation risk assessment

1. Inadequate competencies and training of staff undertaking anticoagulant duties.
2. Failure to initiate anticoagulant therapy where indicated.
3. Poor documentation of reason and treatment plan at commencement of therapy.
4. Prescribed wrong dose or no dose of anticoagulant (especially loading doses).
5. Unconsidered co-prescribing and monitoring of interacting drugs.
6. Unsafe arrangements and communication at discharge from hospital, including failure to adequately transfer duty of care to patient's general practitioner.
7. Insufficient support and monitoring of warfarin therapy for the first 3 months and for vulnerable groups.
8. Inadequate safety checks at repeat prescribing and repeat dispensing in the community.
9. Confusion over anticoagulant management for dentistry, cardioversion, endoscopy and surgical procedures.
10. Potential confusion due to different strength tablets often presented in non-colour-coded packs.
11. The Yellow book (patient-held information), in need of revision and translation into other languages.
12. Inflexible medicine presentation and arrangements in care homes to implement anti-coagulant dose changes.
13. Inadequate quality assurance (QA) for near-patient testing equipment.
14. Inadequate audit of anticoagulant services and/or failure to act on identified risks.

Evidence of disparities between how clinicians think patients are taking warfarin and what patients are actually taking comes from a series of studies by Schillinger and colleagues. In a study with 220 patients taking warfarin the researchers measured (1) adherence by asking patients to report any missed doses and (2) concordance between patients' and providers' reports of warfarin regimens (Schillinger *et al.*, 2006). Patients were categorized as having regimen adherence if they missed no doses, and concordance was defined as patient–provider agreement on weekly dosage. Poor adherence was associated with under-anticoagulation, but not over-anticoagulation. Under-anticoagulation creates significant risk of preventable stroke. Half of the patients (110) reported regimens discordant with their clinicians' report. There was no relationship between patients' reports of adherence and concordance. Among adherent patients, discordance was associated with both underanticoagulation and overanticoagulation. These findings show frequent divergence between patients and the prescriber of their warfarin about what the current dosage regimen was. The researchers recommended that clinicians should separately determine and discuss adherence and regimen with the patient.

The NPSA recommended that, from 1 April, 2008 for patients with a prescription for anticoagulants, community pharmacists in England and Wales should check the following:

Make sure that the patient has a 'yellow book' and that they or their carer understand its contents.

Ask to see patients' latest international normalized ratio (INR) test results in the patient's 'yellow book' before dispensing repeat prescriptions for anticoagulants.

Check that regular INR monitoring is being done.

Where a new medicine is dispensed that might interact with anticoagulants, check that arrangements have been made for additional INR tests.

Pharmacists have been encouraged to record the patient's clinic contact details in their computerized patient medication record. The NPSA recommends that the pharmacist ensures they have a written record of any dosage changes that they obtain in the course of confirming the correct dose (fax or email being acceptable for this purpose). Including this additional step in the therapeutic chain for warfarin should strengthen the safety framework, but the effects of this change are yet to be measured.

The case of diuretics

Diuretics are widely used in hypertension and heart failure and can cause electrolyte and fluid imbalances. A Swedish study of 1600 people aged over 75 found hypokalaemia in 2.5%, hyperkalaemia in 2.8% and hyponatraemia in 9.4% (Passare *et al.*, 2004). Diuretics are not the only medicines involved in electrolyte disturbances but they were a key cause. Hypokalaemia was associated with thiazide-related and combination diuretics; and hyperkalaemia was associated with potassium-sparing diuretics, beta-blockers and tricyclic antidepressants. Hyponatraemia was associated with the use of diuretics, ACE-inhibitors and carbamazepine. Many of the adverse events related to diuretics involve inadequate monitoring of urea and electrolytes (U&Es). A recent French study found no monitoring after more than a year of treatment in 23% of patients aged over 75 and taking diuretics (Gerardin-Marais *et al.*, 2008), as typified by the following account:

Extract from investigation of a complaint made by the patient's daughter:

Mr Y aged 88 years was being treated with furosemide for swelling of the legs. The practice was carrying out monitoring and the most recent test was shown in the records as being done in May of that year. In August Mr Y saw a chiropodist who commented on his swollen feet and recommended that he should see his doctor. Metolazone was added to his treatment. Mr Y's daughter, looking back, commented that her father became increasingly tired, weak and confused. He had several consultations with the practice over the next few months because of his poor health. In January he was visited at home by the Primary care physician and admitted to hospital where he was found to have 'a significant water, sodium and potassium imbalance'. This was the first time his U&Es had been checked since the metolazone was started.

The combination of furosemide with metolazone is well-known to cause electrolyte problems and patients on this combination need frequent checks on U&Es (at least every few weeks).

It is noteworthy that there is no recognized 'gold standard' for frequency of checking U&Es in patients taking diuretics, but good practice might be generally accepted to include:

measuring U&Es one week after starting treatment (and consider doing so again 4–6 weeks after this);

testing 1 week after each dose increase or addition of another diuretic and then at least annually in stable patients;

checking again when another medicine is added that is associated with changes in electrolyte balance (e.g. NSAIDs, ACEIs).

Pharmacists and nurses could play a greater role in ensuring that patients taking diuretics are adequately monitored. Ideally, this would be through access to the part of the patient's record where laboratory test results are recorded. Community pharmacists do not currently have such access, but they and community nurses can ask the patient when they last had a blood test.

The case of NSAIDs

Gastrointestinal adverse events due to NSAIDs have been well known for many years and prescribing and self-medication of NSAIDs remain ubiquitous. Risk factors for NSAID-related adverse events include a history of ulcer disease or bleeding, co-prescribing of medicines that increase propensity for gastric damage or bleeding (corticosteroid, anticoagulant or antiplatelet therapy), and self-medicating with additional NSAIDs (including low-dose aspirin). Older people are more likely to experience ADRs from NSAIDs.

There is evidence that patients and members of the public are not necessarily aware of potential harm from NSAIDs. A large US study of people taking NSAIDs on prescription or by self-medication or both found that 60% of those taking NSAIDs OTC were not aware of the risk of side effects (Wilcox *et al.*, 2005). However, when provided with information about risks and benefits of specific treatments patients' choices are not necessarily the same as prescribers. A US study of 100 patients with osteoarthritis of the knee used adaptive conjoint analysis to explore treatment preferences in the light of information on risks and benefits (Fraenkel *et al.*, 2004). In decreasing order of preference the choices were capsaicin, glucosamine, opioids, non-selective NSAIDs and Cox II inhibitors. The study excluded paracetamol because it was assumed all patients would have tried it already.

There are several interfaces where there is potential to reconsider whether NSAID use might create risk and whether other treatments might be safer. Nurses and pharmacists can ask the following:

1.   Is there any reason to think that it might be better if this patient did not take an NSAID? (Do they have a previous history of ulcer disease or bleeding, are they on corticosteroids, anticoagulant or antiplatelet therapy? Are they in an older age group and more likely to be affected by NSAID adverse effects.)
2.   Does this patient need to take an NSAID, either on prescription or over the counter? (Has paracetamol been discussed and tried at an effective dose and frequency?)
3.   If the patient needs to take an NSAID and is at risk from adverse events, are they being prescribed gastroprotective therapy?

If patients understood better the risk of gastric bleed, they might better avoid this outcome. Clinicians often refer to NSAIDs as 'painkillers' and, while the reason for this shorthand is understandable, it may preclude discussion on the nature, benefits and potential harms of the treatment. More discussion is needed with patients about, for example, why it is important to take the NSAID with food, what 'counts' as food, and help with choosing the most appropriate time to take the NSAID.

The case of antiplatelet medicines

There is significant evidence that low-dose aspirin is effective in preventing cardiovascular events. It also brings increased risk for major gastro-intestinal tract bleeding and a small, but non-significant, increase in the risk for haemorrhagic stroke. Co-prescribing with NSAIDs and SSRIs increases the risk of adverse events. If there is a history of ulcer disease or upper-gastro-intestinal tract bleeding, *Helicobacter pylori* should be eradicated (if present) and a proton pump inhibitor used with aspirin therapy. Pharmacists and nurses can look for, and ask about, these risk factors and risk reduction methods.

Possible solutions

In this section we consider possible ways in which safer medication could be achieved by addressing different points in the processes. The medicines pathway in Fig. 6.1 shows some of the transitions that occur in the prescribing, dispensing, use and monitoring of medicines.

Possible solutions to medication safety issues can be considered in relation to communication at each of the transition points in the medicines pathway. A further framework to guide the design of possible solutions is the principles of good medicines management, which were set out in the Department of Health's 2004 resource on this subject:

1.   Involving patients in the choice of treatment.
2.   Monitoring for benefits.

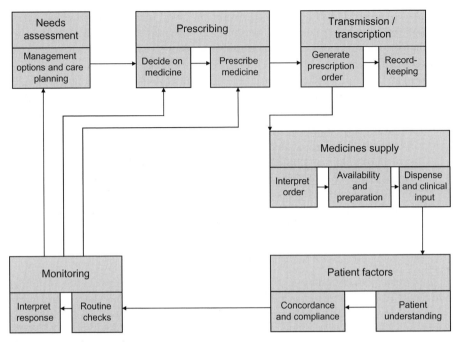

Figure 6.1. Medicines pathway.
Source: Seal, R. National Prescribing Centre 2008 (Clyne *et al.*, 2008).

3. Deciding whether a medicine is still needed.
4. Reviewing effectiveness of treatment.
5. Deciding when to stop a treatment.
6. Reducing medicines wastage.
7. Identifying over- and under-treatment.
8. Making best use of resources – evidence-based formularies and guidelines.
9. Better communications between prescribers, patients and carers.
10. Providing patient-centred information.
11. Consideration of non-pharmacological options, e.g. health promotion, advice, etc.

Source: Department of Health (2004). Management of medicines: a resource to support implementation of wider aspects of medicines management for the National Service Frameworks.

Make monitoring more pro-active in partnership with patients

Monitoring of treatment and long-term conditions tends to be seen as something that is the responsibility of general practice, the more so since the introduction of the Quality and Outcomes Framework (QOF). However, monitoring should be everybody's business in the drive to improve medication safety. Nurse specialists and community pharmacists have key roles to play in discussing, informing, supporting and assisting in an accessible and non-judgemental way. Case managers and community matrons have taken on the role of case managing patients with complex combinations of long-term conditions (Jester, 2007).

It is important not to assume that someone else has already checked that the medicine has been safely prescribed. Some nurses and pharmacists may be hesitant to challenge a doctor's prescription. One reason is likely to be inequitable access to patient's data such that the nurse or pharmacist is insufficiently sure of the justification for their query. Differential professional power is another likely contributor and some pharmacists and nurses may be concerned about adverse consequences from questioning a doctor's decision.

Patients who are fully engaged in their own healthcare are more likely to note, report and discuss any side effects, work together with prescribers to test and identify optimal dosage for that individual patient and to be open about any choices they make to reduce or cease usage of any prescribed medicine. There is a satisfaction for patients to be more in control of their health/symptoms. Involved patients, working in partnership with HCPs, should be less likely to experience an ADR, since they will know about and understand their medicines and use them appropriately.

Make best use of medicines reviews

Medicines reviews are frequently conducted in primary care by GPs, nurses and pharmacists. Table 6.1 from the *Guide to Medication Review* sets out the different types of review and their purpose (Clyne, 2008).

Medicines Use Review (MUR) was introduced in the new community pharmacy contract for England and Wales in 2005 with a focus on whether and how medicines are being used, and patients' understanding of their medicines. MURs are now provided by over 60% of pharmacies and there are, as yet, no data on outcomes. So far, MURs have had little effect on inter-professional working between community pharmacists and general practice (Blenkinsopp *et al.*, 2007). The 2008 Pharmacy White Paper stated the Department of Health's intention that MURs should be more clearly targeted at patient need, and that audit should be conducted (DH, 2008). Pharmacists and local practices could designate patients taking anticoagulants, diuretics, NSAIDs, and antiplatelet medicines as priorities to have an MUR. Working together, practices could share information on test results with local pharmacies and monitor these patients more actively.

Medication review (sometimes referred to as clinical medication review) is undertaken by Primary care physicians, nurses and pharmacists and focuses on clinical aspects of treatment and the patient's condition/s. Ideally conducted face to face with the patient and with access to the patient's records, the review provides an opportunity to bring together information on treatment and test results with the patient's perspective on their health and medicine taking. A face-to-face review provides the perfect opportunity to engage and involve the patient in their own healthcare and to encourage the taking of responsibility for reporting side effects or non-adherence. Experts have recently suggested that, for elderly people '*it is prudent to reassess a patient's entire drug regimen at least twice a year, including categories often overlooked by patients and doctors: drugs bought over the counter and "nutraceuticals" such as herbal remedies or dietary supplements*' (Avorn & Shrank, 2008).

Both MUR and medication review can be targeted at 'moments in care' of transition across interfaces, for example, following patient discharge, or when a new treatment is

Table 6.1. Characteristic of types of medication review

	Purpose of the review	Requires patient to be present	Access to patient's notes	Includes all prescription medicines	Includes prescription, complementary and OTC medicines	Review of medicines and/or condition	Mapping to professional activities
Type 1 **Prescription review**	Address technical issues relating to the prescription e.g. anomalies, changed items, cost-effectiveness	Possibly (any resulting changes to prescribed medicines need to involve the patient)	Yes	Possibly (a prescription review may relate to one therapeutic area only rather than all prescribed medicines)	No	Medicines	• QOF • MUR (prescription intervention)
Type 2 **Concordance and compliance review**	Address issues relating to the patient's medicine-taking behaviour	Possibly (medicines use review by community pharmacist may not include access to patient's notes)	Usually	Yes	Yes	Medicines use	• QOF • MUR • DRUM
Type 3 **Clinical medication review**	Address issues relating to the patient's use of medicines in the context of their clinical condition	Yes	Yes	Yes	Yes	Medicines and condition	• QOF

Remember, the different types of review are not hierarchical but each has a distinct purpose.

initiated. Further guidance on good practice can be found in the National Prescribing Centre's Guide to Medication Review (Clyne, 2008).

Strengthening patient knowledge

Information

The only information that every patient consistently receives about their medicine is the manufacturer's patient information leaflet (PIL). Widely criticized over the years for not being patient-centred, PILS in the EU have been subject to a requirement for user testing since late 2005 (Connelly, 2005). A recent systematic review of medicines manufacturers' patient information leaflets found that medicines information which was tailored to the particular illness was highly valued and that patients want written information to supplement, not substitute for, spoken information from clinicians (Raynor et al., 2007). The same review found widespread ambivalence among clinicians about providing written information to patients, with some favouring only partial disclosure of information on potential harms. The user-friendliness of PILs is generally accepted to have improved since the introduction of user testing. However, PILs do not meet patients' needs for information about medicines in the context of their condition.

The **Department of Health White Paper 'Our health, our care, our say' made a commitment to** '*give all people with long-term health and social care needs and their carers an "information prescription". The information prescription will be given to people using services and their carers by health and social care professionals (for example, GPs, social workers and district nurses) to signpost people to further information and advice to help them take care of their own condition*' (DH, 2006). During 2007–8 20 pilots of Information Prescriptions were conducted to explore how they might be provided in different settings and by different people. The findings will be used to decide how to deliver Information Prescriptions in the future.

Patients themselves are using developments in technology to continue the philosophy of sharing experience and helping each other. The technologies called 'social media' that people use for social networking, entertainment and education are being applied increasingly to health by people with long-term conditions (Sarasohn-Kahn, 2008). See, for example, the MySpace CURE DiABETES group or the DiabetesMine blog. In the past many clinicians have tended towards negativity about patients using the internet for health information and support but will need to reassess their views in the light of recent and future developments. A challenge will be quality assurance to ensure that information is of high quality and accurate and is not provided for commercial purposes.

Self management training

It is principally patients with long-term health conditions who are keen to work in partnership with HCPs and want to self-manage their conditions. The Expert Patient Programme (available in England and Wales) provides a 6-week training programme for those with a range of conditions and some disease-specific versions, as well as courses for carers and parents. Modules include symptom and pain management, relaxation, and communicating with healthcare professionals. Recent statistics from the EPP show that programme graduates make fewer visits to their Primary care physician or A&E, and have an 18% increase in their visits to community pharmacists. Diabetes has seen a major change in the availability of self-management training in recent years with national availability of NHS-resourced DAFNE (dietary adjustment for normal eating) and DESMOND courses. Self-management of anticoagulation has received increasing attention in recent years. For those patients willing and able to learn how to self-manage, a systematic review showed improved quality of oral anticoagulation with improved benefits and reduced harms (Heneghan *et al.*, 2006).

'Know Your Numbers'

The 'Know Your Numbers (KYN)' concept is intended to raise public awareness and knowledge of their own relevant health numbers. These might relate to blood test results and to other measurements including blood pressure and Body Mass Index. Knowledge and understanding of the importance and relevance of specific tests, together with what the number means, could contribute to improved patient safety. Some organizations are promoting KYN including the National Kidney Federation and the Blood Pressure Association. The National Kidney Federation website includes information on different blood tests and normal ranges with a patient-held 'Know Your Numbers' card available for downloading for patients to record their results (NKF, 2008).

Greater use of IT

In addition to the use of social media by patients and carers to share learning about long-term conditions, healthcare providers are also exploring the use of new technologies.

SMS text messaging is being used to send test results and regular reminders about compliance with treatment (for example, weekly bisphosphonates).

A web-based system (MedCheck) was tested, in which patients registered with three primary care medical practices were sent an electronic message 10 days after being prescribed a medicine. MedCheck asked if the patient had filled the prescription or experienced medication-related problems, and then forwarded the patient's response to their primary care physician (Weingart *et al.*, 2008). Of 267 patients studied, 79% opened their MedCheck message and 12% responded to it; 77% responded within 1 day. Patients reported problems filling their prescriptions (48%), problems with drug effectiveness (12%), and medication symptoms (10%). Clinicians responded to 68% of patients' messages; 93% did so within 1 week. Clinicians often supplied or requested information (19%), or made multiple recommendations (15%). Patients experienced 21 total ADEs; they reported 17 electronically.

In the future, general practice computer systems will have greater capability to identify preventable medicines-related problems. The PRIMIS project has developed a specification for software that would at least partly address many of the issues identified in this chapter. In the meantime, better human communication has the capacity to improve medication safety.

Conclusions

We know from research the types of medicines-related problems that occur at interfaces in the healthcare system and the reasons why they happen. Clinicians (both prescribing and non-prescribing) need to work more closely together and with patients to deal with the well-recognized problems. Clinicians should not make assumptions that someone else in the system has checked or confirmed that it is safe for a medicine to be used and need to be more pro-active and to take greater responsibility for their role in ensuring safety.

Possible solutions include working in partnership with patients, including pro-active monitoring, more effective use of medicines reviews and strengthening patient knowledge.

References

Avorn J, Shrank WH. (2008). Adverse drug reactions in elderly people: a substantial cause of preventable illness. *British Medical Journal*, **336**, 956–7.

Baglin TP, Cousins D, Keeling DM, Perry DJ, Watson HG. (2006). Recommendations from the British Committee for Standards in Haematology and National Patient Safety Agency. *British Journal of Haematology*, **136**, 26–9.

Blenkinsopp A, Celino G, Bond CM, Inch J. (2007). Medicines Use Review: The first year of a new community pharmacy service. *Pharm Journal*, **278**, 218–23.

Chen YF, Neil KE, Avery AJ, Dewey ME, Johnson C. (2005). Prescribing errors and other problems reported by community pharmacists. *Therapy Clinical Risk Management*, **1**(4), 333–42.

Clinical Knowledge Service. Patient Leaflet. Anti-inflammatories non-steroidal. http://www.cks.library.nhs.uk/patient_information_leaflet/anti_inflammatories_non_steroidal (accessed 17/5/09).

Clyne W, Blenkinsopp A, Seal R. (2008). A guide to medication review. NPC Plus with Medicines Partnership. http://www.npci.org.uk/medicines.management/review/medireview/library/librarygoodpracticeguide1.Php. Accessed 30/3/09.

Connelly D. (2005). User testing of PILs now mandatory. *Pharm J 2005*; **275**, 12.

Fraenkel L, Wittink D, Concato J, Fried T. (2004). Treatment options in knee osteoarthritis: the patient's perspective. *Archives Intemat Medicine, ***164**, 1299–304.

Gérardin-Marais M, Victorri-Vigneau C, Allain-Veyrac G, *et al.* (2008). Diuretic drug therapy monitoring in the elderly: a cohort study. *European Journal of Clinical Pharmacology*, **64**, 433–7.

Hansen LB, Fernald D, Araya-Guerra R, Westfall JM, West D, Pace W. (2006). Pharmacy clarification of prescriptions ordered in primary care: a report from the Applied Strategies for Improving Patient Safety (ASIPS) collaborative. *Journal of the American Board Family Medicine*, **19**(1), 24–30.

Heneghan C, Alonso-Coello P, Garcia-Allemina JM, Perera R, Meats E, Glasziou P. (2006). Self-monitoring of oral anticoagulation: a systematic review and meta analysis. *Lancet*, **367**, 404–11.

Howard R, Avery A, Bissell P. (2008) Causes of preventable drug-related hospital admissions: a qualitative study. *Quality and Safety in Health Care*, **17**, 109–16.

Howard RL, Avery AJ, Slavenburg S, *et al.* (2007). Which drugs cause preventable admissions to hospital? A systematic review. *British Journal of Clinical Pharmacology*, **63**(2), 136–47.

Indermitte J, Beutler M, Bruppacher R, Meier CR, Hersberger KE. (2007). Management of drug-interaction alerts in community pharmacies. *Journal of Clinical Pharm Therapy*, **32**(2), 133–42.

Jester R. (2007). In: *Advancing Practice in Rehabilitation Nursing*. Blackwell Publishing (2007).

Moberly T. (2008). Community pharmacy plays its part in making anticoagulation safer. *Pharm Journal*, **280**, 78.

National Kidney Federation. Know Your Numbers. http://www.kidney.org.uk/

Medical-Info/other/know_nos.html (accessed 28/4/08).

National Patient Safety Agency. (2008). Anticoagulant therapy: information for community pharmacists.

Passare G, Viitanen M, Törring O, Winblad B, Fastbom J. (2004). Sodium and potassium disturbances in the elderly: prevalence and association with drug use. *Clinical Drug Investigation*, **24**(9), 535–44.

Raynor DK, Blenkinsopp A, Knapp P, *et al.* (2007). A systematic review of quantitative and qualitative research on the role and effectiveness of written information available to patients about individual medicines. *Health Technol Assessment*, (**5**):iii, 1–160. Review.

Sarahsohn-Kahn J. (2008). The wisdom of patients. Healthcare meets online social media. California Health Foundation. http://www.chcf.org/documents/chronicdisease/HealthCareSocialMedia.pdf (accessed 28/4/08).

Schillinger D, Wang F, Rodriguez M, Bindman A, Machtinger EL. (2006). The importance of establishing regimen concordance in preventing medication errors in anticoagulant care. *Journal of Health Communications*, **11**(6), 555–67.

Spinewine A. (2008). The challenge of safer prescribing. *British Medical Journal*, **336**, 956–7.

Weingart SN, Gandhi TK, Seger AC, *et al.* (2005). Patient-reported medication symptoms in primary care. *Archives Intern Medicine*, **165**(2), 234–40.

Weingart SN, Hamrick HE, Tutkus S, *et al.* (2008). Medication safety messages for patients via the web portal: The MedCheck intervention. *Int J Med Inform*, **77**(3), 161–8.

Wilcox CM, Cryer B, Triadafilopoulos G. (2005). Patterns of use and public perception of over-the-counter pain relievers: focus on nonsteroidal antiinflammatory drugs. *Journal of Rheumatology*, **32**(11), 2218–24.

Witherington EM, Pirzada OM, Avery AJ. (2008). Communication gaps and readmissions to hospital for patients aged 75 years and older: observational study. *Quality Safety Health Care*, **17**(1), 71–5.

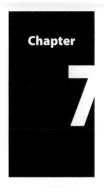

Parenteral drug administration

Jasmeet Soar and Jon Standing

Introduction

Parenteral drug administration refers to drugs given by routes other than the digestive tract. The term parenteral is usually used for drugs given by injection or infusion. The enteral route usually refers to taking drugs by mouth. The common parenteral routes are listed in Table 7.1. In the USA the Food and Drug Administration (FDA) lists over 100 routes of drug administration (www.fda.gov/cder/dsm/).

Most hospital patients receive parenteral drugs at some time during their stay. Parenteral drug use is also increasingly common in the community setting (O'Hanlon, 2008). The intravenous (IV) route is associated with errors in several stages of the medication process (prescribing, preparing and administration) and this route has been associated with a higher number of errors than any other route (Hunt & Rapp, 1996; Cousins *et al.*, 2005).

In one hospital ward study, there was at least one error made during preparation and administration in 212 (49%) out of 430 intravenous drug doses (Taxis & Barber, 2003). It is therefore important to only give drugs parenterally if it is not possible to use the simpler oral route – it is essential that the medication prescription is reviewed regularly and drug treatments changed to the safer oral route at the earliest opportunity.

Reasons for parenteral drug administration

The common reasons for giving drugs parenterally are listed below.

1. The enteral route is not possible. For example, following major abdominal surgery or a critical illness, patients can have delayed gastric emptying or an ileus (Artinyan *et al.*, 2008). In this situation, the enteral route is unreliable until gut function returns to normal.

Table 7.1. Parenteral routes of drug administration

Common parenteral routes of drug administration		
Route	Abbreviation	Examples
Intravenous	IV	IV bolus of cefuroxime over 3 minutes.
		Intermittent infusion of vancomycin over 1 hour once daily according to plasma levels.
		Continuous IV unfractionated heparin infusion.
Intramuscular	IM	IM injection of morphine
Subcutaneous	SC	SC injection of enoxaparin.
		SC infusion of morphine in palliative care.

Medication Safety: An Essential Guide, ed. Molly Courtenay and Matt Griffiths. Published by Cambridge University Press. © M. Courtenay and M. Griffiths 2009.

2. There is a need to rapidly achieve therapeutic plasma levels of the drug and the drug effect. This is why anaesthetic drugs and drugs in life-threatening emergencies (e.g. antibiotics in life-threatening infections, drugs used in cardiac arrest) are mainly given by the IV route (Nolan et al., 2005).

3. The drug is only available as a parenteral preparation. Some drugs are poorly absorbed if given orally (e.g. heparin) or are metabolized by the liver (e.g. the short-acting beta-blocker, esmolol). This results in very little active drug getting into the patient's plasma, and then reaching the drug target site. Drug effects are therefore reduced. Drugs that do not work after being taken orally are said to have poor oral bioavailability.

4. The plasma drug levels need to be rapidly and carefully adjusted to avoid over- or under-dosing, i.e. drugs with a narrow therapeutic index and rapid onset and offset of action. An intravenous infusion enables careful titration of the drug to achieve the desired effect. Each of the following requires monitoring of the drug effect and adjustments of the drug infusion.

   - Noradrenaline infusions are adjusted to achieve a target blood pressure in critically ill patients in the intensive care unit.
   - Heparin infusions are titrated to maintain the activated partial thrombo-plastin time (APTT). The APTT is a measure of the blood's ability to clot and becomes prolonged after heparin infusion. Too much heparin can excessively prolong the APTT and this increases the risk of uncontrolled bleeding.
   - Short-acting insulin is infused IV to maintain a normal blood sugar.

Some drugs are given parenterally for a combination of these reasons.

Problems with parenteral drug administration

In the UK, the National Patient Safety Agency (NPSA) received 14 228 reports of incidents associated with injectable medicines between January 2005 and June 2006 (National Patient Safety Agency, 2007). This accounted for 2.2% of the total number of incidents reported to the NPSA and 24% of all the medication incidents reported. Twenty-five (0.2%) injectable medication incidents resulted in patient death and 28 (0.2%) in severe patient harm. The common reasons for these incidents are listed in Table 7.2. It is important to realize that the NPSA reporting scheme relies on voluntary reports and that the actual number of patients being harmed by errors associated with injecting parenteral drugs is likely to be far higher. How these problems can be avoided will be covered in the remainder of this chapter.

Methods of parenteral drug administration

The nature of the drug determines the precise route by which a medicine will be administered parenterally. In general, IV drugs have a faster onset of action than intramuscular (IM) drugs, which, in turn, have a faster onset of action than subcutaneous (SC) drugs. These parenteral routes tend to work faster than the oral route. Intravenous drugs go directly into the venous circulation. IM and SC drugs rely on local absorption into

Table 7.2. Injectable medicines incidents reported between January 2005 and June 2006

Type of incident	Percentage of events (total = 14 228)
Wrong dose, strength or frequency	28.9
Omitted medicine/ingredient	14.4
Wrong drug	10.2
Wrong quantity	8.7
Wrong route	5.1
Wrong/transposed/ omitted medicine label	3.3
Wrong formulation	3.2
Patient allergic to treatment	3.0
Wrong patient	2.9
Adverse drug reaction	2.8
Others	17.5

Based on data from the National Patient Safety Agency (National Patient Safety Agency, 2007).

the circulation. This will depend on local tissue blood flow and is more variable and less reliable than the IV route.

Intravenous drug administration

Intravenous drug administration requires the patient to have a venous catheter. There are a wide variety of venous catheters, often referred to as vascular access devices (VADs). The commonest types of VADs (Gabriel, 2008a, b) are:

1. peripheral venous cannulae;
2. central venous catheters (CVCs);
3. peripherally inserted central cannulae (PICCs).

Peripheral venous cannulae

Most IV drugs are given through a peripheral venous cannulae inserted into the back of the hand or forearm. Peripheral cannulae have a limited duration of use. Peripheral cannulae should not be used for more than 72 hours as this increases the risk of infection, blockage or extravasation of drugs.

Central venous catheter

Central venous catheters (CVCs) have their tip positioned in the superior vena cava just above the right atrium. They are usually inserted into the right side of the neck through the internal jugular vein or through the subclavian vein. CVCs deliver drugs through large central veins as these medicines are irritable to peripheral veins or can cause severe tissue damage if they extravasate (e.g. noradrenaline, chemotherapy drugs). Drugs given through a central vein will have a faster onset of action than drugs given through a peripheral vein. This is because they are given closer to the heart, and are rapidly pumped into the systemic circulation to their target sites.

CVCs can have more than one lumen (e.g. triple lumen) and this enables several infusions to be given at the same time. CVCs are associated with a greater risk on insertion (pneumothorax, bleeding) and are prone to infection (McGee & Gould, 2003). Newer CVCs are available that are coated with silver or antibiotic combinations that claim to decrease the risk of related infections (Gilbert & Harden, 2008). Patients who require IV drug therapy over a number of months (e.g. chemotherapy) or long-term parenteral nutrition require the insertion of a tunnelled central venous catheter (e.g. Hickman® line, Groshong® line). The Epic 2 - National Evidence-Based Guidelines for Preventing Healthcare-Associated Infections in NHS hospitals in England provide detailed guidance on the insertion, use and removal of central venous catheters (Pratt et al., 2007).

Peripherally inserted central cannulae (PICC)

There is increasing use of PICC lines for long-term use as they are technically easier to insert. These lines are inserted through an arm vein and threaded so that the tip lies in the superior vena cava. Some recent studies question whether PICCs offer any real benefit to patients over central venous catheters for long-term use (Cowl et al., 2000; Turcotte et al., 2006). 'Midlines' are a variation of the PICC line. These devices are shorter and the tip of the line is in the axillary vein.

Infusion systems

Drugs can be injected from a syringe by hand or infused using an infusion device. Infusion devices require specific training in their use. Ideally, all infusion devices should be standardized in a clinical setting to simplify education in their use. In the UK, the Medicines and Healthcare products Regulatory Agency (MHRA) has produced specific guidance on the safe use of infusion systems (www.mhra.gov.uk). All infusion systems should be checked regularly during infusion (e.g. hourly).

Common devices used for intravenous infusion include the following:

1. **Syringe pumps** (Fig. 7.1). These enable controlled delivery of the drug from a syringe (usually at 0.1 to 99.9 ml/h). Some syringe pumps have other functions such as patient controlled analgesia (PCA) (Viscusi, 2008). These can be programmed to enable the patient to administer an IV dose of analgesic (usually morphine). The programme ensures the patient only receives a single dose over a defined period ('lockout') irrespective of the number of times the patient presses the button. Bedside pumps often have a key guard to prevent tampering with the syringe, and password protection, so they can only be reprogrammed by a trained person.

Although syringe drivers are limited by the volume of drug they can infuse and the infusion rate, they have the advantage of portability over volumetric infusion pumps (see below). It is essential that the correct type and make of syringe is used for a particular pump to ensure correct drug infusion rates. Newer infusion pumps will give the user prompts that ensure all the information entered is correct before the infusion is started. Infusion pumps should be placed at the level of the patient. Having a pump positioned at a higher level can cause errors by increasing the rate of infusion (Neff et al., 2001; Donald et al., 2007).

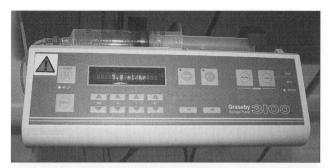

Figure 7.1. Syringe infusion pumps.

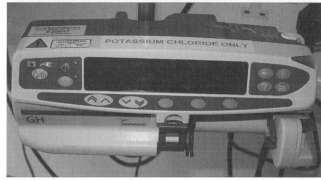

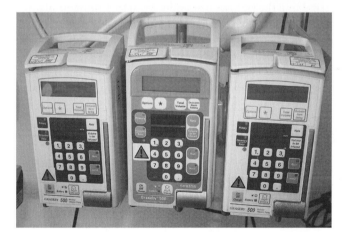

Figure 7.2. Volumetric infusion pumps.

2. **Volumetric pumps** (Fig. 7.2). These are mainly used for larger volume infusions (e.g. IV fluid therapy) at a rate of 1 to 999 ml/h. These pumps require specific administration sets that vary between manufacturers.

Intramuscular (IM) drug administration

The commonest site for IM injection is the anterolateral aspect of the middle of the patient's thigh. Alternatives include the deltoid muscle (upper arm) or the now less commonly used upper outer quadrant of the buttock (gluteal route) (Wynaden *et al.*, 2005). There is a risk of damage to the sciatic nerve when medicines are given by the

Table 7.3. Needle gauges and lengths

Standard UK needle gauges and lengths		
Brown	26 G	10 mm
Orange	25 G	16 mm or 25 mm
Blue	23 G	25 mm
Green	21 G	38 mm

Department of Health (2006).

gluteal route (Small, 2004). It is important to follow the drug manufacturer's instruction for the optimum site for IM injection. Manufacturers will provide information regarding the best site for IM injection to achieve a response.

For IM injections, the needle needs to be long enough to ensure that the drug is injected into the muscle (Table 7.3). For injections into the thigh area, a 25 mm needle is best (e.g. blue needle – 25 mm and 23 G) and is suitable for all ages. In pre-term or very small infants, a 16 mm needle is suitable for IM injection. In some adults, a longer length (38 mm) may be required. For gluteal injections a much longer needle is often required (Zaybak *et al.*, 2007).

Subcutaneous (SC) drug administration

A SC injection is administered into the fat layer just under the skin. Common sites for SC injections are the upper outer arm, the thighs and the abdomen. The skin should be pinched and the injection given with the needle at a 45° or 90° angle to the skin. An orange needle (16 mm and 25 G) is suitable for SC injections.

It is common in palliative care settings to give analgesic and sedative drugs (e.g. midazolam and diamorphine) by continuous subcutaneous infusion using a syringe driver (Costello *et al.*, 2008).

Practicalities of parenteral drug administration

Prescribing of parenteral drugs

Prescriptions for parenteral medicines must be written clearly without any ambiguity. Prescription details required are described in Box 7.1.

For complex prescriptions (e.g. heparin infusion and insulin sliding scales), it is best to have standardized prescription charts as this will minimize deviations from best practice. When patients are on multiple parenteral drugs or complex drug regimens, the prescription chart should be reviewed regularly (ideally daily) by a pharmacist. This is especially important when prescriptions are for children.

Preparation and checking of drugs for administration

A number of factors need to be considered when preparing and checking medicines for administration. The following is based on guidance from the University College Hospitals pharmacy department (University College Hospital, 2007) and the National Patient Safety Agency (National Patient Safety Agency, 2007).

Box 7.1 Prescribing information

Patient details (name, hospital number, date of birth or address)
Allergies or previous adverse drug reactions
Date and time of administration
Approved full name of injectable medication
Dose and frequency
Route of administration
Diluent and volume if infusion needs to be reconstituted
Information to calculate dose, e.g. patient weight, coagulation screen for heparin infusion rate
Review date/time for the prescription
Finish date/time or maximum number of doses
Prescriber's signature – legible so that it can be identified

- Drugs should ideally be prepared immediately before use by the person administrating them. Some drugs are available ready prepared, and labelled in prefilled syringes (e.g. adrenaline prefilled syringes for cardiopulmonary resuscitation, low molecular weight heparins).
- It is essential that the individual giving the drug understands the following:
  - How the drug is reconstituted.
  - How to calculate the dose, concentration of the final solution and rate of infusion – example calculations for complex drugs or infusion charts should be available in clinical areas to minimize calculation errors (Wright, 2008).
  - The compatibility of the drug with diluents (e.g. 0.9% saline or 5% dextrose) and other drugs (e.g. in administration tubing, at Y-connectors or three-way taps).
  - The stability of the drug – drugs infusions should not be left in a syringe for longer than recommended by the drug manufacturer. For continuous infusions, the syringe should be changed at regular intervals according to local policy (e.g. every 24 hours or less if there is a specific recommendation).
  - Whether the drug can be injected as a bolus by hand or requires to be infused over a set period. This is important as some drugs have side effects when given rapidly (e.g. vancomycin causes flushing, i.e. red man syndrome) or can cause pain on IV injection (e.g. cyclizine, erythromycin).
  - If there is a need for special handling or precautions (e.g. to be kept out of the light or avoid temperature fluctuations).
- Information about the drug can be checked with the medications summary of the product characteristics (SPC).
- Hands should be washed before preparing the drug. The drug should be prepared on a clean surface and gloves worn. In general, non-sterile gloves can be used as long as syringe and injection ports remain untouched during an IV injection. Local guidelines must be followed. In some hospitals sterile gloves must be worn when administrating drugs through a central venous catheter.
- Drugs should be prepared and checked in a quiet area without distraction to minimize errors during preparation.
- Ensure drugs are properly mixed – some drugs can layer and require thorough mixing (e.g. potassium chloride and 5% dextrose – potassium chloride is denser

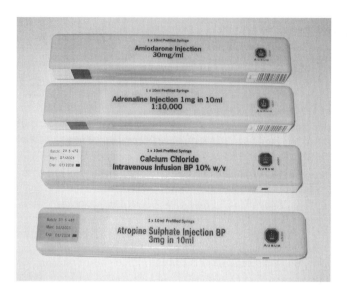

Figure 7.3. Drugs with similar sounding names or similar packaging.

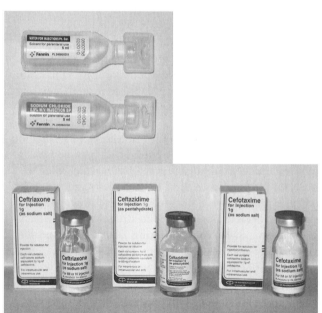

and sinks to the bottom of the container). Other drugs need to be mixed slowly to avoid foaming (e.g. teicoplanin and water).

- Read the drug labels carefully and check the expiry date. Some drug preparations can look very similar. Also similar drug names (Lambert *et al.*, 2005) and packaging (Kenagy & Stein, 2001) can cause confusion (Fig. 7.3).
- All syringes or infusion bags should be labelled immediately following reconstitution (Fig. 7.4). Unlabelled syringes can lead to drug errors. The syringe volume markings should not be obscured by the label.

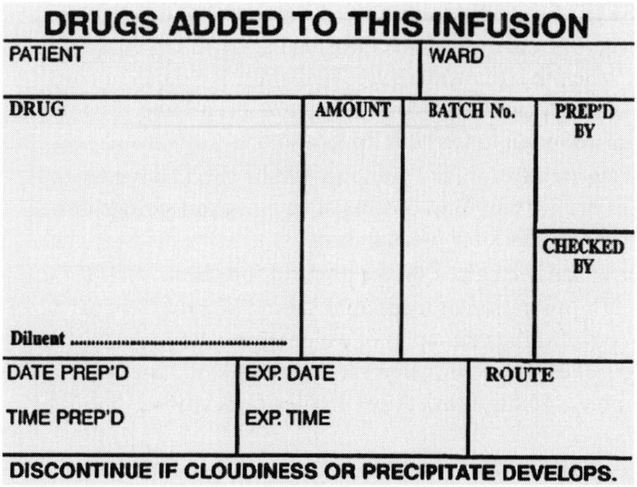

DRUGS ADDED TO THIS INFUSION

PATIENT			WARD	
DRUG		AMOUNT	BATCH No.	PREP'D BY
				CHECKED BY
Diluent				
DATE PREP'D	EXP. DATE		ROUTE	
TIME PREP'D	EXP. TIME			

DISCONTINUE IF CLOUDINESS OR PRECIPITATE DEVELOPS.

Figure 7.4. Drug label.

- Drugs should be checked against the prescription to ensure the correct dose of the correct drug is given at the correct time to the correct patient.
- The prepared drug, empty drug ampoules or vials, diluent ampoules, and prescription charts should be taken in a clean tray to the patient for immediate administration.
- The patient should be identified verbally and visually by checking their name band against the prescription chart.
- It should be ensured that the patient is not allergic to the drug by checking the drug chart and talking to the patient.
- The patient should be provided with an explanation of what you are going to administer and why. All medicines licensed in the UK will have a patient information leaflet available.
- A final check of the prescription chart, drugs and patient should be undertaken prior to administering the drug.
- For IV drugs, IV access needs to be checked to confirm it is working. This can be checked by injecting 0.9% saline or 5% dextrose first.
- An aseptic non-touch technique (ANTT) should be used to deliver the drug.
- The patient should be monitored after giving the drug, i.e. to look for an expected effect of the drug (e.g. decrease in blood glucose after insulin) or an adverse effect (e.g. anaphylactic reaction – see below).
- Ampoules and needles should be disposed of in a sharps container. Injectable medicines should be for single use only unless the label specifically indicates that they are licensed and suitable for multi-dosing.
- When using infusion devices, ensure that they are plugged into the main electricity supply at the patient bedside, or have an adequate battery supply if being used during patient transfer.
- When two drugs are infused IV simultaneously into the same vein it is essential to ensure that both drugs are infused into the patient at the required rate (e.g.

paired infusion of 10% glucose and insulin for a sliding scale). If the venous catheter is occluded, there is a danger of one infusion backtracking up the second infusion line. When the occlusion is resolved, there is a danger of an accidental bolus of the drug that has backtracked up the second line. This can be avoided by using an infusion pump for both drugs and one-way valves.

- If the patient is receiving an infusion, the pump should be checked regularly to monitor the amount of drug given. The contents of any infusion syringe or bag should also be monitored to check for precipitation.
- Document that the drug has been given on the prescription chart.
- Staff involved in the administration of medicines should be proficient at calculations, and understand the principles of weight per volume percentages (e.g. 1% w/v = 10 mg/ml) as well as infusion rates (e.g. 100 ml 3 mg/ml solution over 30 minutes = 10 mg/min). Any complex calculations should be double checked.
- Injectable cytotoxic drugs should be supplied to clinical areas ready to use and specifically labelled. These drugs should only be used in specified areas and administered by individuals who have had specific training in cytotoxic drug administration.
- If there are any queries, advice should be sought from senior colleagues or a pharmacist.

Flushing between drugs and venous catheter locks

Venous catheters should be flushed before giving an IV drug, in-between giving different IV drugs, and after giving an IV drug.

- Flushing a catheter before giving a drug ensures the catheter is working correctly.
- Flushing a venous catheter in-between giving two different drugs will prevent incompatible drugs mixing and precipitating.
- Flushing after giving an IV drug ensures there is no drug left inside the catheter. There is a risk that this will result in an accident bolus of any residual drug left in the catheter (the volume of space inside the catheter is often called the dead space volume) the next time the venous catheter is used. This is especially important with central venous catheters, which can have a large dead space volume, and in children where a small bolus of a residual drug is at greater risk of causing a harmful effect.

The commonest choice of flush is 0.9% sodium chloride (normal saline) or 5% dextrose – check with the drug information to ensure that the drugs being administered are compatible with the flush solution. Peripheral IV cannulae need a flush volume of 5–10 ml, whereas central venous catheters require larger flush volumes (e.g. 20 ml). It is important to infuse the flush at the same rate as the original drug being administered. This will prevent the patient getting an accidental rapid bolus of the original drug.

Specialist advice should be sought regarding flush volumes for neonatal venous devices – these flush volumes tend to be in the order of 1–2 ml.

It is common to flush venous cannulae that are not in use. This prevents the cannulae becoming blocked (e.g. 0.9% sodium chloride IV flush, 8 hourly). Ideally, venous cannulae that are not being used should be removed to minimize risk of infection, unless they are being kept for a specific reason.

For central venous catheters, it is common to fill the dead space of the catheter with a lock solution (e.g. heparin, citrate, antibiotic). This prevents the catheter from getting blocked by blood clots and prevents infection. The volume of the lock must be accurately known so that when the lock is injected into the catheter, it only reaches the catheter tip and does not go into the patient's bloodstream. Catheters containing locks should be carefully labelled so that the next person using the catheter removes the lock drug prior to catheter use.

Specific hazards of intravenous drug administration

Needle stick injury to individuals administering drug

Staff must minimize the risk of needle stick injury. Needle-free injection systems or blunt needles for drawing up drugs should be used wherever possible. Needles should be disposed in a 'sharps' container. The most serious risks associated with needle stick injuries are Hepatitis B virus (HBV), Hepatitis C virus (HCV) and Human immuno-deficiency virus (HIV) (Tarantola *et al.*, 2006). HBV vaccination is recommended for all healthcare workers (unless they are immune to this virus because of previous exposure). No vaccine exists to prevent HCV or HIV infection. In the event of a needle stick injury, it is essential that occupational health services are contacted immediately to ensure correct treatment. Individuals who have a needle stick injury and are at risk of HIV infection may be offered anti-retroviral drug therapy (PEP – post-exposure prophylaxis) (Young *et al.*, 2007).

Drug extravasation

Drug extravasation occurs when a drug given intravenously leaks out into the surrounding tissues ('the cannulae has tissued')(Hadaway, 2007). The risk of harm depends on the drug injected and can include pain, reddening of the skin and, with certain drugs, skin ulceration and necrosis. Drugs that are particularly irritant or damaging if they extravasate should be given through a central venous line (e.g. vaso-constrictors: adrenaline, noradrenaline, some cytotoxic drugs, drugs with a high or low pH or an osmolarity greater than plasma (>290 mosmol/l)). Extravasation needs to be dealt with urgently to prevent tissue necrosis. In this situation, the following steps should be taken:

- Leave the cannulae in situ.
- Try to aspirate any drug through the cannulae using a syringe – this may not work but is worth trying.
- Elevate the patient's limb.
- Look at the drug data sheet for specific instructions and seek expert advice. For example, there is a specific antidote (dexrazoxone) for extravasation of the cytotoxic anthracycline.

Anaphylaxis after parenteral drug administration

Anaphylaxis is a severe, life-threatening, generalized or systemic hypersensitivity reaction

This is characterized by rapidly developing life-threatening airway and/or breathing and/or circulation problems usually associated with skin and mucosal changes (Soar *et al.*, 2008).

There are approximately 20 anaphylaxis deaths reported each year in the UK, although this may be a substantial under-estimate. When anaphylaxis is fatal, death usually occurs very soon after contact with the trigger. Deaths caused by IV drugs occur most commonly within 5 minutes.

Anaphylaxis is likely when all of the following three criteria are met:

- sudden onset and rapid progression of symptoms;
- life-threatening airway and/or breathing and/or circulation problems;
- skin and/or mucosal changes (flushing, urticaria, angioedema).

The following supports the diagnosis:

- exposure to a known allergen for the patient (Soar *et al.*, 2008).

Remember:

- skin or mucosal changes alone are not a sign of an anaphylactic reaction;
- skin and mucosal changes can be subtle or absent in up to 20% of reactions (some patients can have only a decrease in blood pressure, i.e. a circulation problem);
- There can also be gastro-intestinal symptoms (e.g. vomiting, abdominal pain, incontinence).

Skin and/or mucosal changes

These should be assessed as part of the **Exposure** when using the ABCDE approach.

- They are often the first feature and present in over 80% of anaphylactic reactions.
- They can be subtle or dramatic.
- There may be just skin, just mucosal, or both skin and mucosal changes.
- There may be erythema – a patchy, or generalized, red rash.
- There may be urticaria (also called hives, nettle rash, weals or welts), which can appear anywhere on the body. The weals may be pale, pink or red, and may look like nettle stings. They can be different shapes and sizes, and are often surrounded by a red flare. They are usually itchy.
- Angioedema is similar to urticaria but involves swelling of deeper tissues, most commonly in the eyelids and lips, and sometimes in the mouth and throat.

Although skin changes can be worrying or distressing for patients and for those treating them, skin changes without life-threatening airway, breathing or circulation problems do not signify an anaphylactic reaction.

There can be confusion between an anaphylactic reaction and a panic attack. Victims of previous anaphylaxis may be particularly prone to panic attacks if they think

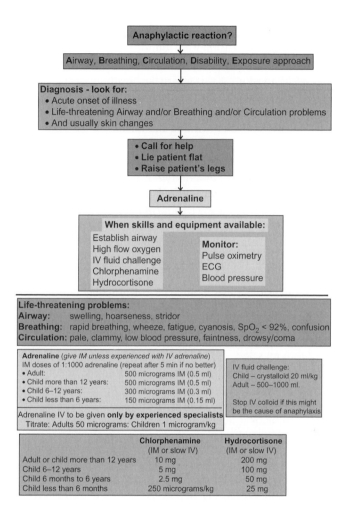

Figure 7.5. Anaphylaxis algorithm (reproduced with permission from the Resuscitation Council UK).

they have been re-exposed to the allergen that caused a previous problem. The sense of impending doom and breathlessness leading to hyperventilation are symptoms that resemble anaphylaxis in some ways. While there is no hypotension, pallor, wheeze, or urticarial rash or swelling, there may sometimes be flushing or blotchy skin associated with anxiety, adding to the diagnostic difficulty. Diagnostic difficulty may also occur with vasovagal attacks after immunization procedures. However, the absence of rash, breathing difficulties and swelling are useful distinguishing features, as is the slow pulse of a vasovagal attack compared with the rapid pulse of a severe anaphylactic episode. Fainting will usually respond to lying the patient down and raising the legs.

The treatment of anaphylaxis is summarized in the anaphylaxis algorithm (Fig. 7. 5)

- As the diagnosis of anaphylaxis is not always obvious, all those who treat anaphylaxis must use the systematic Airway, Breathing, Circulation, Disability,

Exposure (ABCDE) approach when dealing with the sick patient. Any life-threatening problems should be treated as they are found.

- All patients should be placed in a comfortable position. Patients with airway and breathing problems may prefer to sit up as this will make breathing easier. Lying flat with or without leg elevation is helpful for patients with low blood pressure (circulation problem). If the patient feels faint, do not sit or stand them up – this can cause cardiac arrest. Patients who are breathing and unconscious should be placed on the side (recovery position).

- Drug suspected of causing an anaphylactic reaction should be stopped (e.g. intravenous infusions of a gelatin solution or antibiotic). Definitive treatment should not be delayed if removing the trigger is not feasible.

- Adrenaline is the most important drug for the treatment of an anaphylactic reaction. Adrenaline seems to works best when given early after the onset of the reaction, but it is not without risk, particularly when given intravenously. The intramuscular (IM) route is the best for most individuals who have to give adrenaline to treat an anaphylactic reaction. Monitor the patient as soon as possible (pulse, blood pressure, ECG, pulse oximetry). This will help monitor the response to adrenaline.

- The best site for IM injection is the anterolateral aspect of the middle third of the thigh. The needle used for injection needs to be sufficiently long to ensure that the adrenaline is injected into muscle.

- The IV route for adrenaline must only be used by those expert in the use of adrenaline in their every day practice (e.g. intensivists). Most rescuers should use the IM route.

- Antihistamines are a second-line treatment for an anaphylactic reaction. Corticosteroids may help prevent or shorten protracted reactions.

Reporting drug errors and adverse events

Drug administration errors should be reported so that future similar incidents can be prevented. Although most healthcare staff are in agreement that drug errors should be reported, many do not report errors when they occur. Healthcare settings should have drug error reporting systems and action plans in place to prevent the same errors occurring repeatedly. In the UK, adverse drug reactions should be reported to the MHRA using the Yellow Card scheme (www.mhra.gov.uk). The *British National Formulary (BNF)* also includes copies of the Yellow Card at the back of each edition.

References

Artinyan A, Nunoo-Mensah, Balasubramaniam JWS, *et al.* (2008). Prolonged postoperative ileus-definition, risk factors, and 'predictors after surgery'. *World Journal of Surgery*, **32**(7), 1495–500.

Costello J, Nyatanga B, Mula C, Hull J. (2008). The benefits and drawbacks of syringe drivers in palliative care. *International J Palliative Nursing*, **14**(3), 139–44.

Cousins DH, Sabatier B, Begue D, Schmittownal AC, Hope-Tichy T. (2005). Medication errors in intravenous drug preparation and administration: a multicentre audit in the UK, Germany and France.

Quality and Safety in Health Care, **14**(3), 190–5.

Cowl CT, Weinstock JV, Al-Jurf A, Ephgrave K, Murray JA, Dillon K. (2000). Complications and cost associated with parenteral nutrition delivered to hospitalized patients through either subclavian or peripherally-inserted central catheters. *Clinical Nutrition*, **19**(4), 237–43.

Department of Health UK, *Immunisation Against Infectious Disease*. 2006.

Donald AI, Chinthamuneedi MP, Spearritt D. (2007). Effect of changes in syringe driver height on flow: a small quantitative study. *Critical Care Resusc*, **9**(2), 143–7.

Gabriel J. (2008a). Infusion therapy. Part 1: Minimising the risks. *Nursing Standard*, **22**(31), 51–6; quiz 58.

Gabriel J. (2008b). Infusion therapy. Part 2: Prevention and management of complications. *Nursing Standard*, **22**(32), 41–8; quiz 50.

Gilbert RE, Harden M. (2008). Effectiveness of impregnated central venous catheters for catheter related blood stream infection: a systematic review. *Current Opinion in Infectious Diseases*, **21**(3), 235–45.

Hadaway L. (2007). Infiltration and extravasation. *American Journal of Nursing*, **107**(8), 64–72.

Hunt ML, Jr, Rapp RP. (1996). Intravenous medication errors. *Journal of Intravenous Nursing*, **19**(3 Suppl), S9–15.

Kenagy JW, Stein GC. (2001). Naming, labeling, and packaging of pharmaceuticals. *American Journal of Health Systems in Pharmacy*, **58**(21), 2033–41.

Lambert BL, Lin SJ, Tan H. (2005). Designing safe drug names. *Drug Safety*, **28**(6), 495–512.

McGee DC, Gould MK. (2003). Preventing complications of central venous catheterization. *New England Journal of Medicine*, **348**(12), 1123–33.

National Patient Safety Agency. *Patient Safety Alert 20: Promoting*

Safer Use of Injectable Medicines. March 2007.

Neff TA, Fischer JE, Schulz G, Baenziger O, Weissm M. (2001). Infusion pump performance with vertical displacement: effect of syringe pump and assembly type. *Intensive Care Medicine*, **27**(1), 287–91.

Nolan JP, Deakin CD, Soar J, Bottiger BW, Smith G. (2005). European Resuscitation Council guidelines for resuscitation 2005. Section 4. Adult advanced life support. *Resuscitation*, **67** Suppl. 1, S39–86.

O'Hanlon S. (2008). Delivering intravenous therapy in the community setting. *Nursing Standard*, **22**(31), 44–8.

Pratt RJ, Pellowe CM, Wilson JA. (2007). epic2: National evidence-based guidelines for preventing healthcare-associated infections in NHS hospitals in England. *Journal of Hospital Infection*, **65** Suppl. 1, S1–64.

Small SP. (2004). Preventing sciatic nerve injury from intramuscular injections: literature review. *Journal Advanced of Nursing*, **47**(3), 287–96.

Soar J, Pumphrey R, Cant A, *et al.* (2008). Emergency treatment of anaphylactic reactions – guidelines for healthcare providers. *Resuscitation*, **77**(2), 157–69.

Tarantola A, Abiteboul D, Rachine A. (2006). Infection risks following accidental exposure to blood or body fluids in health care workers: a review of pathogens transmitted in published case. *American Journal on Infection Control*, **34**(6), 367–75.

Taxis K, Barber N. (2003). Ethnographic study of incidence and severity of intravenous drug errors. *British Medical Journal*, **326**(7391), 684.

Turcotte S, Dube S, Beauchamp G. (2006). Peripherally inserted central venous catheters are not superior to central venous catheters in the acute care of surgical patients on the ward. *World Journal of Surgery*, **30**(8), 1605–19.

University College Hospitals Pharmacy Department. *Injectable Medicines Administration Guide*. 2nd edition (2007). Oxford, UK: Blackwell Publishing.

Viscusi ER. (2008). Patient-controlled drug delivery for acute postoperative pain management: a review of current and emerging technologies. *Regional Anesthesia and Pain Medicine*, **33**(2), 146–58.

Wright K. (2008). Drug calculations part 1: a critique of the formula used by nurses. *Nursing Standard*, **22**(36), 40–2.

Wynaden D, Landsborough I, Chapmen R, McGowan S, Lapsley J, Finn M. (2005). Establishing best practice guidelines for administration of intramuscular injections in the adult: a systematic review of the literature. *Contemporary Nurse*, **20**(2), 267–77.

Young TN, Arens FJ, Kennedy GE, Laurie JW, Rutherford G. (2007). Antiretroviral post-exposure prophylaxis (PEP) for occupational HIV exposure. *Cochrane Database Systems Review*(1), CD002835.

Zaybak A, Gunes UY, Tamsel S, Khorshid L, Eser I. (2007). Does obesity prevent the needle from reaching muscle in intramuscular injections? *Journal of Advanced Nursing*, **58**(6), 552–6.

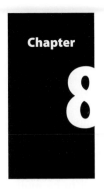

8 Calculations

Alison G. Eggleton

Introduction

In his report 'Building a safer NHS for patients: Improving medication safety' (DH, Smith, 2004), the Chief Pharmaceutical Officer (CPO), Dr Jim Smith, recognized calculation error as a key risk factor in the medication process. According to Lesar (1998), the most common preventable adverse drug events occur due to errors in prescribing of medicines, and of these more than 15% are due to errors in the use of dosing equations. The National Patient Safety Agency (NPSA) defines a complex calculation as one where more than one step is required for preparation and/or administration of a medicine (NPSA, 2007b). Examples quoted include infusions where the dose is quoted in micrograms/kg per hour or where there is a need for dose unit conversion such as milligram to millimole or percentage to milligram.

Inadequacies in the ability of healthcare professionals to perform calculations accurately have been widely reported. Wheeler *et al.* (2004), for example, reported that registered doctors had difficulties with drug dosage calculations, particularly when the strengths of solution were expressed as ratios or percentages. A further report (Wheeler *et al.*, 2007) identified that newly qualified doctors and those working in community practice struggled significantly more, as well as those from certain medical schools.

The dispensing of a defective medicine, which led to the death of a 3-week-old baby (peppermint water containing an excessive amount of chloroform) by a pre-registration pharmacy trainee and a pharmacist qualified for 21 months, resulted in an increased emphasis on calculation skills training for pharmacists by the Royal Pharmaceutical Society of Great Britain (RPSGB, 2007–08). Pharmacy pre-registration trainees must attain at least 70% in 20 calculation questions as part of the final examination before registration and pre-registration tutors must specifically comment on trainees' progress in calculation skills through their quarterly appraisal reports (RPSGB, 2007-08).

Sabin (2003) identified, through a literature review, a lack of proficiency within the nursing profession, both amongst students and registered practitioners, and made 11 recommendations for future practice. These included the assessment of competence in calculations to include both the acquisition of mathematical knowledge and its application within actual clinical practice. The Nursing and Midwifery Council (NMC, 2004) requires that entrants to pre-registration nursing programmes have numeracy skills sufficient to ensure proficiency in drug calculation skills relevant to professional requirements. This definition of proficiency may vary according to the sector of practice. For example, in paediatrics complex drug calculations are commonplace and a 100% passmark in the assessment may be required (Sandwell & Carson, 2005).

Medication Safety: An Essential Guide, ed. Molly Courtenay and Matt Griffiths. Published by Cambridge University Press. © M. Courtenay and M. Griffiths 2009.

Similarly, in the 'Standards of proficiency for nurse and midwife prescribers', the NMC recommends a pass mark of 100% in the calculation assessment for independent nurse prescribers (NMC, 2006).

Geissler (in Sabin, 2003) suggests that the issues of calculation competence raised regarding the nursing profession apply equally to other healthcare professions. Thus the importance of good calculation skills amongst healthcare professionals has become widely accepted. Sabin (2003) says that calculation efficacy is not only influenced by mathematical ability as evidenced by qualifications. Errors tend to be multifactorial and additionally are affected by factors such as knowledge of the medication(s), length of experience of the practitioner, shift patterns, workload, staffing levels and the quality of the written prescription itself. Gender may also have a role, since females are thought more likely to have a negative attitude towards, and therefore feel anxious about, mathematics. Kohn *et al.* (2000) argued that the people employed in healthcare are generally well educated and dedicated, and do not intend harm to their patients. They advocate a systems-based approach to risk management because errors are more often due to the convergence of multiple contributing factors rather than the failure of an individual. In addition to improving competence in calculation skills, therefore, healthcare systems must be made safer so that the risk of error is reduced. In line with this approach, the NPSA (2007b) recommended several risk reduction strategies in relation to high-risk injectable medicines. Ready-to-use products should be sourced and used whenever possible. However, when such a product is unavailable, the risk may be minimized by methods such as the provision of dose calculating tools, guidance on prescribing, preparation and administration and the provision of pre-printed prescriptions.

The CPO (DH, 2004) listed several common sources of calculation error including:

- prescribing of potent medicines;
- prescribing for children.

The 'Institute for Safe Medication Practices' (ISMP, 2007a) published a list of high-alert medications that carry a greater risk of causing significant harm to patients if used in error, although mistakes in the use of these drugs are not necessarily more common. In this chapter, we will look at basic calculation skills within the context of commonly reported errors. Suggestions will also be made as to how systems may be improved to reduce the risk of calculation errors. Drugs from the high-alert medicines list will be used in the worked examples where possible.

Dosage units

The system of measurement used in the UK is the metric system. In prescribing of medicines, probably the most commonly used units are those of mass and volume. Mass is more commonly referred to as weight and the basic metric unit is the gram (g). The basic metric unit of volume is the litre (l). Drug amounts are also commonly referred to in terms of a base unit called a mole (mol). However, it is common for multiples or fractions of these base units to be used. It is essential, therefore, that healthcare professionals understand the terminology around units of measurement and are able to convert between different dosage units. Failure to do so can result in an error of large magnitude, such as 1000-fold.

Prefixes

There are three prefixes commonly used in the UK metric system:

- *kilo* meaning one thousand times greater than the base unit. For example: a kilogram is 1000 grams.
- *milli* meaning one thousand times less than the base unit. For example: a milligram is a 1000th of a gram.
- *micro* meaning one million times less than the base unit. For example; a microgram is a 1 000 000th of a gram.

Units of volume

The units of volume are the litre (l) and millilitre (ml). One litre is equivalent to 1000 millilitres. To convert a volume in litres into a volume in millilitres, multiply the number of litres by 1000. To convert a volume in millilitres into litres, divide the number of millilitres by 1000.

For example:

Example. Convert 2.5 l into millilitres.

Volume in millilitres $= 2.5 \, l \times 1000$
$= 2500 \, ml$

To check that you have done this calculation correctly, you can imagine moving the decimal place. To multiply by 1000, you have to move the decimal place three places to the right.

2.5 x 1000 = 2 . 5 0 0

= 2500 ml

Example. Convert 1750 ml into litres.

Volume in litres $= 1750 \, ml \div 1000$
$= 1.75 \, l$

To check that you have done this calculation correctly, you can imagine moving the decimal place. To divide by 1000, you have to move the decimal place three places to the left.

1750 ÷ 1000 = 1 7 5 0 .

= 1.75 l

Units of mass

The units of weight (or mass) are the gram (g), the kilogram (kg), the milligram (mg), the microgram and, less commonly, the nanogram.

The units of weight are related to each other as shown in Table 8.1. Because there is a 1000-fold difference between each of these units, a mistake in their use can result in a catastrophic error. For example, a pre-term infant died following the administration of a parenteral nutrition solution containing an overdose of zinc. The concentration of zinc had inadvertently been entered into the pharmacy computer for an automatic compounding system at a final concentration of 330 mg/100 ml instead of 330 micrograms/100 ml (ISMP, 2007b).

To convert from the larger unit of weight into the next unit down in Table 8.1, multiply by 1000.

For example:

Example. Convert 4.5 kg into grams.

Weight in grams = 4.5 kg × 1000

= 4500 g

To check that you have done this calculation correctly, you can imagine moving the decimal place. To multiply by 1000, you have to move the decimal place three places to the right.

$$4.5 \times 1000 = 4 . 5 \quad 0 \quad 0$$

$$= 4500\,g$$

Example. Convert 7.5 g into milligrams.

Weight in milligrams = 7.5 g × 1000

= 7500 mg

Example. Convert 250 mg into micrograms.

Weight in micrograms = 250 mg × 1000

= 250 000 micrograms

Table 8. 1. Units of mass

Unit	Abbreviated to	Equivalent to
1 kilogram	kg	1000 g
1 gram	g	1000 mg
1 milligram	mg	1000 micrograms
1 microgram		1000 nanograms

Example. Convert 5 micrograms into nanograms.

Weight in nanograms = 5 micrograms × 1000
= 5000 nanograms

To convert from the smaller unit of weight into the next larger unit in Table 8.1, you must divide by 1000.

For example:

Example. Convert 500 micrograms into milligrams.

$500 \div 1000 = 0.5$ mg

To check that you have done this calculation correctly, you can imagine moving the decimal place. To divide by 1000, you have to move the decimal place three places to the left.

$$500 \div 1000 = \qquad 5 \quad 0 \quad 0 \,.$$

$$= 0.5mg$$

Example. Convert 250 mg into grams.

250 mg $\div 1000 = 0.25$ g

Example. Convert 2500 g into kilograms.

$2500 \div 1000 = 2.5$ kg

Example. Convert 250 nanograms into milligrams.

$250 \div 1000 = 0.25$ mg

Units of amount

The term used for the base unit of the amount of a drug is called a *mole*, usually expressed as a mass or weight. One mole of a substance is the molecular, atomic or ionic weight of the substance expressed in grams. So, for example, one mole of sodium chloride (NaCl) would be the weight of one sodium ion (23) plus the weight of one chloride ion (35.5) expressed in grams, a total of 58.5 g. A molar solution is one which contains one mole of a substance dissolved in one litre of fluid. So, for example, a molar aqueous solution of sodium chloride contains 58.5 g in 1 litre of water. The term *millimole* (meaning a 1000th of a mole) is used commonly in biochemistry results. For example, a serum potassium concentration might be stated as 3.5 mmol/l.

The term 'normal' saline, or more correctly physiological saline, is sodium chloride solution 0.9%. This means it contains 0.9 g sodium chloride in 100 ml, or 9 g in a litre. The next example shows how to work out the number of millimoles of sodium and chloride in a litre of 'normal' saline.

Example 1

One mole of sodium chloride is 58.5 g.

A molar solution of sodium chloride contains 58.5 g in 1 l.

Therefore, a solution containing 9 g sodium chloride per litre contains:

$$9 \div 58.5 \times 1 \text{ mole} = 0.153 \text{ mole}$$

Convert this to millimoles by multiplying by 1000.

$$0.153 \text{ mole} \times 1000 = 153 \text{ mmol}$$

Therefore, one litre of a 'normal' saline contains 153 mmol sodium ions and 153 mmol chloride ions. In practice, this is commonly rounded down and stated as 150 mmol per litre of sodium and of chloride ions.

Safety tips

Explicit policies should be in place in each healthcare organization to ensure that only agreed standardized abbreviations are used (Expert Group on Safe Medication Practices, 2006). The terms 'microgram' and 'nanogram' should always be written in full and not abbreviated, particularly if written by hand (BMA and RPSGB, 2007). This is because the abbreviations that have been used ('mcg' or 'μg' for microgram, and 'ng' for nanogram) have led to drug errors when they have been misread as mg for milligram (ISMP, 2000). Similarly, the abbreviation 'u' should never be used to replace 'unit' because a badly written 'u' can be read as a zero, leading to a 10-fold overdose, or as a four, leading to a 4-fold overdose (ISMP, 1997; ISMP, 2008; NPSA, 2007a).

An individual practitioner may make what is termed an *endogenous* error because of a random and unpredictable cognitive event. If, for example, one practitioner made an error such as a dose miscalculation, a second practitioner performing the same calculation would not often make the same error. An endogenous error is more likely to be detected if there is a double-check performed by a second person *as a separate independent action* (ISMP, 2003; NPSA, 2007b). Therefore, where a calculation is performed, it should *always* be checked independently by a second individual, ideally by another doctor, nurse or pharmacist. This is particularly important if the calculation involves a high-risk drug such as chemotherapy (Smith, 2004), a high-risk patient group such as neonates or children (Hutton & Gardner, 2005), or a high-alert medicine (ISMP, 2007a). If the calculation is checked independently, without looking at the first person's work, the second person is less likely to be misled into the same faulty thinking that led to the original error (ISMP, 2003).

The need for dosage calculations by staff should be minimized through a systems-based approach (ISMP, 2003). For example, standard medicine concentrations, standard dosing charts or validated protocols should be developed for situations where calculations would otherwise be regularly required. Solutions, medicine concentrations, doses and administration times should be standardized whenever possible (Expert Group on Safe Medication Practices, 2006). Ready-to-use and ready-to-administer preparations should be actively sought, purchased and used whenever possible to avoid the need for dose calculation and/or multiple manipulations in the preparation of a product (NPSA, 2007b).

Walton *et al.* (1999) reviewed comparative studies where computer programs were used to advise doctors on appropriate drug dosage. Drugs involved included many high-alert medicines (ISMP, 2007a) such as midazolam, fentanyl, lidocaine, warfarin and heparin, and drugs requiring therapeutic drug monitoring (theophylline, aminoglycosides). Computer assistance was shown overall to benefit patient care and reduce unwanted effects of treatment. However, even where dose calculators are developed, the need for a second check must not be overlooked. For example, the 'Livingston Paediatric Dose Calculator' was published to assist with paediatric drug dosing in emergency departments, but the authors still recommended a double-check of calculated doses (Reed & Fothergill, 2007). Errors in the dosage of several drugs in the dose calculator were highlighted, leading to the publication of a revised version (Weatherup, 2007). Independent validation of such tools is essential before publication, as well as a revision date to ensure currency.

Test yourself with practice calculations

Before you continue, test yourself with these calculations to make sure you have understood this section. Answers are given at the end of this chapter.

1. Try converting the following amounts:
   (a) How much is 0.5 kg in grams?
   (b) How much is 62.5 mg in micrograms?
   (c) How much is 250 micrograms in milligrams?
   (d) How much is 3500 ml in litres?
   (e) How much is 1.75 l in millilitres?

Understanding concentrations

Amount per volume

The usual method of expressing the concentration of a liquid preparation is an amount per unit volume. For example:

> micrograms per millilitre (micrograms/ml)
> milligrams per millilitre (mg/ml)
> millimoles per litre (mmol/l)
> grams per litre (g/l)

These expressions are required when calculating the volume of a solution required to administer a specified dose to a patient.

Example 1

How would a dose of 125 micrograms of digoxin be given to a patient from an ampoule of digoxin injection containing 500 micrograms in 2 ml?

Step 1: calculate the amount of digoxin in 1 ml of solution. Solution contains 500 micrograms in 2 ml. Therefore, it contains 500 micrograms ÷ 2 = 250 micrograms in 1 ml

Step 2: the volume of solution that would contain 125 micrograms is:

$$\frac{125}{250} \times 1 \text{ ml} = 0.5 \text{ ml}$$

Example 2

How would a dose of 2.5 mg of midazolam be given to a patient from an ampoule of midazolam injection containing 10 mg in 2 ml?

Step 1: calculate the amount of midazolam in 1 ml of solution. Solution contains 10 mg in 2 ml. Therefore, it contains 10 mg ÷ 2 = 5 mg in 1 ml.

Step 2: calculate the volume of solution that contains 2.5 mg midazolam. Solution contains 5 mg in 1 ml. Therefore, for a dose of 2 mg, we would need:

$$\frac{2.5}{5} \times 1 \text{ ml} = 0.5 \text{ ml}$$

It is recommended that the practitioner estimates what a sensible answer would be before carrying out the actual calculation so that a mistake would be more likely to be identified (Hutton & Gardner, 2005). So, in Example 2 above, if the ampoule contains 10 mg in 2 ml, and you want to give a 2.5 mg dose, then your answer *must* be a smaller amount that 2 ml. Once the calculations become more complex, and perhaps involve several steps, this ability to estimate the answer becomes even more important. Similarly, if a calculator is used, the practitioner should always check if the answer makes common sense. Errors can easily occur when entering data into a calculator, and the temptation is simply to accept the answer without question. Using a calculator does not replace a basic understanding of the mathematics underpinning the calculation.

Some people like to think of the calculations in Examples 1 and 2 as the formula:

$$\frac{\text{Dose required}}{\text{Strength available}} \times \text{volume} = \text{volume required}$$

OR

$$\frac{\text{What you want}}{\text{What you've got}} \times \text{volume} = \text{volume required}$$

Look at Example 3 below.

Example 3

We want to give a child a dose of morphine sulphate 3 mg (what you want) from a solution containing 10 mg in 5 ml (what you've got). How do we calculate the volume required?

$$\frac{3 \text{ mg}}{10 \text{ mg}} \times 5 \text{ ml} = \text{volume required (ml)}$$

Therefore, the volume required to give a 3 mg dose is 1.5 ml.

To estimate if you have the right answer, think about this logically. If your solution contains morphine sulphate 10 mg in 5 ml, it must contain 5 mg in 2.5 ml, or 2.5 mg in 1.25 ml. Therefore, to give a dose of 3 mg (which lies between 2.5 mg and 5 mg), your answer must lie between 1.25 ml and 2.5 ml. If it does not (for example, if you had the figures in the calculation the wrong way round), your answer would not make sense and you would know you had made a mistake. The best way to become familiar with this type of calculation, with or without the help of a calculator, is to practise with simple calculations to which you know the answer (Hutton & Gardner, 2005).

Percentage concentrations

Some manufacturers express the concentration of their product as a percentage. A percentage is the amount of ingredient in 100 parts of the product. In other words, to calculate a percentage, put the figure over 100.

For example, if you have sodium chloride 1.8% solution, this means it is

$$\frac{1.8 \text{ g}}{100 \text{ ml}}$$

Percentage concentrations can be found in both solid and liquid preparations. You will see the following types of percentage expressions in Table 8.2.

Example 4

How much magnesium sulphate is contained in 5 ml of magnesium sulphate 50% injection?

Step 1: work out what the percentage strength means in grams per 100 ml. Magnesium sulphate 50% injection contains 50 g magnesium sulphate in 100 ml solution.

Step 2: calculate how much magnesium sulphate there is in 5 ml of the solution.

$$\frac{5}{100} \times 50 \text{ g} = 2.5 \text{ g}$$

Concentrations expressed in ratios or parts

A ratio is often used to describe the concentration of very dilute solutions. It expresses the number of grams of a drug that are dissolved or dispersed in a given number of parts of a solution in millilitres. For example, adrenaline solution 1 in 1000 contains 1 g adrenaline in 1000 ml of solution. Because these solutions tend to be very dilute and yet very potent, it is important to take great care with these calculations.

Example 5

How much adrenaline is contained in 1 ml of adrenaline 1 in 1000 solution?
Step 1: work out what the ratio strength means.

Adrenaline 1 in 1000 = 1 g in 1000 ml

Table 8.2. Percentage expressions

% w/v	This describes a percentage weight in volume. The weight will be in grams and the volume in millilitres. For example: sodium bicarbonate 4.2% w/v solution contains 4.2 g sodium bicarbonate in 100 ml solution
% w/w	This describes a percentage weight in weight, most commonly of a solid. Both weights will be in grams. For example: betamethasone 0.1% w/w cream contains 0.1 g betamethasone in 100 g cream
% v/v	This describes a percentage volume in volume of a liquid. Both volumes will be in millilitres. For example, liquid paraffin oral emulsion 50% v/v contains 50 ml liquid paraffin in 100 ml emulsion

Step 2: convert the strength of the solution to milligrams.

1g in 1000 ml = 1000 mg in 1000 ml

Step 3: calculate how much adrenaline there is in 1 ml of the solution.

$$\frac{1}{1000} \times 1000 = 1 \text{ mg in 1 ml}$$

Example 6

How much adrenaline is contained in 10 ml of adrenaline 1 in 10 000 dilute solution?

Step 1: work out what the ratio strength means.

Adrenaline 1 in 10000 = 1 g in 10000 ml

Step 2: convert the strength of the solution to milligrams.

1 g in 10 000 ml = 1000 mg in 10 000 ml

Step 3: calculate how much adrenaline there is in 10 ml of the solution.

$$\frac{10}{10\,000} \times 1000 = 1 \text{ mg in 10 ml}$$

Safety tips

Several authors have reported an increased likelihood of drug dose calculation errors when strengths of solutions are expressed as ratios or percentages (Scrimshire, 1989; Rolfe and Harper, 1995; Wheeler *et al.*, 2004; Wheeler *et al.*, 2007) leading to calls for standardization of labelling to mass concentration. Indeed, the standardization of methods for labelling, packaging and storing medicines is a key safety objective within the Expert Group on Safe Medication Practices report (2006). Apkon *et al.* (2004) described a systems-based approach to risk reduction in a paediatric intensive care setting. The intravenous drug infusion process was characterized into key elements by a multidisciplinary team, and then each stage revised to improve reliability. Standardization of drug formulations and development of dose calculators were two of the methods employed to reduce risk to patients. Wheeler *et al.* (2006) showed that additional on-line teaching of medical students improved knowledge about drug administration, although this waned over time and required reinforcement. Wheeler *et al.* (2007) advocated the formal teaching and testing of drug administration skills both in medical school and in the training of newly qualified doctors. Competence in calculation skills should be taught to healthcare professionals during training, and continuously be reinforced after registration.

Test yourself with practice calculations

Before you continue, test yourself with these calculations to make sure you have understood this section. Answers are given at the end of the chapter.

1. The dose of propofol to induce anaesthesia in an adult aged less than 55 years is 1.5–2.5 mg/kg. Your patient weighs 70 kg and you decide to give a dose of

1.5 mg/kg. Therefore, you require a dose of 105 mg propofol. What volume of propofol 1% injection will contain this dose?

2. You want to give a bolus dose of 100 mg lidocaine to a patient to control ventricular arrhythmia. The injection solution you have is lidocaine injection 2%. What volume of the injection do you need to give this dose?

3. A child aged 6 years requires a dose of propranolol IV of 20 micrograms/kg. The child weighs 20 kg and therefore the total dose needed is 400 micrograms. The injection solution contains 1 mg in 1 ml. What volume of the injection solution is required to give this dose?

4. A child aged 15 years requires a dose of 500 micrograms of adrenaline for acute anaphylaxis (a dose used when there is doubt as to the adequacy of the circulation). The injection solution available is adrenaline 1 in 10 000. What volume of this injection solution is required to administer this dose?

Calculating the dose

The *dose* of a drug is the amount of drug given to the patient to achieve a therapeutic outcome. Dosage calculation is common in certain patient groups such as children, with more potent drugs such as chemotherapy, and with certain types of drug administration including the intravenous route. Therefore, the need for accuracy in calculations is very important. Care must be taken in the interpretation of dosage statements. The dose may be stated as the amount *per dose*. For example, according to the BNF for Children (BMJ, RPSGB, RCPCH, 2008), the usual dose of co-amoxiclav suspension 125 mg in 5 ml for a child aged 1 month to 1 year is 0.25 ml/kg *per dose* and the dose is *repeated three times a day*. Alternatively the dose may be stated as the amount to be given *in total per day*, which then needs to be divided according to the recommended frequency of administration. So, for example, again according to the BNF for Children (BMJ, RPSGB, RCPCH, 2008), the dose of potassium to treat potassium depletion is 1–2 mmol/kg daily in 2–3 divided doses.

Calculated doses may need to be rounded up or down in order to match with availability of a drug formulation. For example, for dissolution of gallstones, the dose of ursodeoxycholic acid in the BNF is 8–12 mg/kg daily as a single dose at bedtime or in two divided doses (BMA, RPSGB, September 2008). For a patient weighing 70 kg, the possible total daily dose range would be 560–840 mg. The product is available as tablets of 150 mg and 300 mg, or capsules of 250 mg. Therefore, there are various options available, such as one 300 mg tablet twice a day (600 mg per day) or three 250 mg tablets together taken at bedtime (750 mg per day).

Dosage calculations can be based on:

- a given amount of drug per kilogram body weight of the patient;
- a given amount of drug based on a patient's body surface area;
- a given rate of drug administration per unit time.

Calculating a dose based on patient's body weight

When a dosage statement is given as an amount *per kilogram body weight*, this means that you have to multiply the amount per dose by the patient's measured or estimated body weight in order to get the total dose to administer. For example, if the dose of a drug is 5 mg/kg, this means you would give 5 mg for every 1 kg of body weight. If the patient weighed 2 kg, the dose would be $(2 \times 5) = 10$ mg. If the patient weighed 20 kg, the dose would be $(20 \times 5) = 100$ mg. You must be very careful to read the dosage statement because it may appear in other units, such as micrograms/kg, or ml/kg, or mmol/kg. The following are some examples:

Example 1

Calculate the dose of liposomal amphotericin for an adult weighing 75 kg. The microbiologist has requested a dose of 3 mg/kg daily as a single daily dose.

Step 1: calculate the dose:

Dose = Patient's weight (kg) × amount per dose (mg/kg)
$$= 75 \text{ kg} \times 3 \text{ mg/kg}$$
$$= 225 \text{ mg}$$

Example 2

Calculate the dose of co-amoxiclav suspension 125/31 in 5 ml for a child aged 6 months weighing 8 kg. The dose is 0.25 ml/kg repeated three times a day.

Step 1: calculate the dose:

Dose = Patient's weight (kg) × amount per dose (ml/kg)
$$= 8 \text{ kg} \times 0.25 \text{ ml/kg}$$
$$= 2 \text{ ml}$$

Therefore, the dose of co-amoxiclav 125/31 in 5 ml suspension would be 2 ml three times a day.

Example 3

Calculate the dose of salbutamol oral solution for a child aged 2 years weighing 12 kg. The dose is 100 micrograms/kg (to a maximum of 2 mg) three to four times a day.

Step 1: calculate dose.

Dose = Patient's weight (kg) × amount per dose (micrograms/kg)
$$= 12 \text{ kg} \times 100 \text{ micrograms/kg}$$
$$= 1200 \text{ micrograms}$$
$$= 1200 \text{ mcg} \div 1000 = 1.2 \text{ mg}$$

Step 2: calculate the volume of salbutamol oral solution that contains 1.2 mg. Salbutamol oral solution contains 2 mg salbutamol in 5 ml.

$$\frac{\text{Dose required}}{\text{Strength available}} \times \text{volume} = \text{volume required}$$

$$\frac{1.2 \text{ mg}}{2 \text{ mg}} \times 5 \text{ ml} = 3 \text{ ml}$$

Therefore, the dose of salbutamol for the child would be 1.2 mg (3 ml of salbutamol syrup 2 mg/5 ml) three to four times a day.

Example 4

Calculate the daily dose of oral potassium chloride required to reverse potassium depletion in a 6-year-old child weighing 20 kg. The dose you require is 2 mmol/kg per day in two to three divided doses. You are going to give the dose using potassium chloride syrup 1 mmol/ml.

Step 1: calculate the total daily dose.

$$\text{Dose per day} = \text{Patient's weight (kg)} \times \text{amount per dose (mmol/kg)}$$
$$= 20 \text{ kg} \times 2 \text{ mmol/kg}$$
$$= 40 \text{ mmol}$$

The total daily dose must be divided into two to three doses, say 20 mmol twice daily.

Step 2: calculate the volume of potassium chloride syrup 1 mmol/ml that contains 20 mmol of potassium.

$$\frac{\text{Dose required}}{\text{Strength available}} \times \text{volume} = \text{volume required}$$
$$\frac{20 \text{ mmol}}{1 \text{ mmol}} \times 1 \text{ ml} = 20 \text{ ml}$$

Therefore, the dose of potassium chloride for the child would be 20 mmol (20 ml of potassium chloride syrup 1 mmol/ml) twice a day.

Dosage calculations can sometimes be based on a patient's ideal body weight rather than actual body weight. The following equations can be used to calculate the ideal body weight.

Male: Ideal body weight = $(0.9 \times \text{height in centimetres}) - 88 \text{ kg}$
Female: Ideal body weight = $(0.9 \times \text{height in centimetres}) - 92 \text{ kg}$

Example 5

Calculate the dose of gentamicin for an adult female patient to treat septicaemia. The microbiologist has advised a single daily dose regime of 5 mg/kg based on ideal body weight. The patient weighs 65 kg and is 160 cm tall. You have gentamicin 40 mg/ml injection available.

Step 1: Calculate the patient's ideal body weight:

$$\text{Female ideal body weight (IBW)} = (0.9 \times \text{height in centimetres}) - 92 \text{ kg}$$
$$= (0.9 \times 160) - 92 \text{ kg}$$
$$= 52 \text{ kg}$$

Step 2: calculate the total daily dose.

$$\text{Daily dose} = \text{Patient's IBW (kg)} \times \text{amount per dose (mg/kg)}$$
$$= 52 \text{ kg} \times 5 \text{ mg/kg}$$
$$= 260 \text{ mg}$$

Step 3: calculate the volume of gentamicin 40 mg in 1 ml injection that contains 260 mg.

$$\frac{\text{Dose required}}{\text{Strength available}} \times \text{volume} = \text{volume required}$$
$$\frac{260}{40} \times 1 = 6.5 \text{ ml}$$

The dose of gentamicin based on ideal body weight would therefore be 260 mg (6.5 ml) of gentamicin injection 40 mg in 1 ml given once a day.

Calculating the dose based on a patient's body surface area

Dosage calculations can be based on the patient's body surface area (BSA) rather than body weight. BSA calculations were originally introduced to work out safe starting doses in the early stages of trials of drugs in humans, which had previously only been tested in animals. They have since become routine practice for dosing of many anti-cancer drugs in adult oncology. They were originally constructed from a very small study (Du Bois & Du Bois, 1916) whose accuracy has since been disputed (Jones *et al.*, 1985; Wang *et al.*, 1992), and neither drug response nor toxicity are necessarily closely related to BSA. In paediatric oncology, dosage is now more commonly calculated from body weight, although BSA nomograms still appear in the BNF for children (BMJ, RPSGB, RCPCH, 2007). Because the BSA calculation method is still widely used in adult oncology, healthcare professionals need to understand it. However, prescribing in oncology is a specialized and high-risk field of practice and policy often dictates that prescribing must be initiated by a consultant or specialist registrar. These calculation examples are merely included to raise awareness of this method of calculating doses. Anyone anticipating working in the field of oncology must ensure that further specialist training in dosage calculation is undertaken.

In general, body surface area is estimated using a nomogram. Prescribers must be careful to select the correct nomogram because different ones are available for adults, children and adolescents and infants. To use the nomogram, you need to know the patient's height in centimetres and weight in kilograms. The nomogram consists of a scale depicting the height, one depicting weight and a third depicting body surface area. The user simply marks the height on one scale, the weight on the second scale and draws a line between the two points. The BSA is then taken as the point at which this line bisects the BSA scale. *The example shown in Fig. 8.1 is not an accurate scale – it merely illustrates the point.*

Example 6

Calculate the dose of cyclophosphamide using the low dose intravenous regimen of 80 mg/m^2 once a week for an adult patient with a body surface area estimated at 1.6 m^2.

Step 1: calculate the dose for a patient with a body surface area of 1.6 m^2.

$$\text{Weekly dose} = 80 \text{ mg/m}^2 \times 1.6 \text{ m}^2$$
$$= 128 \text{ mg}$$

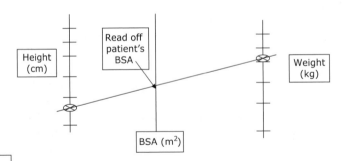

Figure 8.1. Representation of a body surface area calculator (not to scale).

Doses of cytotoxic drugs may be prepared for the individual patient according to BSA or may sometimes be dose banded. Dose banding was introduced as a risk reduction strategy in response to increasing workload in oncology pharmacies. A selection of standard doses is prepared in advance. When a dose is required for a given patient, a selection of pre-prepared syringes is used to make up the dose to within 5% of the patient's calculated dose. Amongst other advantages, this method has been found to reduce calculations and thus the risk of arithmetical and dose calculation errors (MacLean *et al.*, 2003). Cyclophosphamide is one of the drugs described as being suitable for dose banding. Although this method improves workflow and may minimize risk by reducing the need for complex manipulations under pressure during preparation, the accuracy of the original dosage calculation is still of paramount importance.

Test yourself with practice calculations

Before you continue, test yourself with these calculations to make sure you have understood this section. Answers are given at the end of the chapter.

1. What is the ideal body weight of the following patients?
    (a)   A man who is 185 cm tall?
    (b)   A woman who is 150 cm tall?

2. What is the dose of co-amoxiclav suspension 125/35 for a child aged 5 years weighing 18 kg? The dose is 0.25 ml/kg repeated three times a day.

3. Calculate the dose of tobramycin for an adult female to treat a severe infection to be given by slow intravenous bolus injection. The dose recommended in the BNF for a severe infection is 5 mg/kg daily in divided doses every 6 to 8 hours. The dose must be based on ideal body weight. The patient is 165 cm tall. Tobramycin injection contains 40 mg in 1 ml.

4. Calculate the dose of cyclophosphamide using the low dose intravenous regimen for an adult patient with a body surface area estimated at 1.85 m^2. The selected dose is 120 mg/m^2 once a week.

Calculating the rate of drug administration per unit time

For practitioners working in high-risk patient care areas, such as critical care, the calculations in this section are of paramount importance. Calculations of this type unquestionably fall into the NPSA definition of high risk (NPSA, 2007b). In addition, the types of drugs used in critical care areas are frequently high-risk drugs in a clinical sense, for example, inotropic drugs. In the practice situation every effort should be made to reduce and minimize the risk to patients. Practitioners must ensure that validated drug dosage calculators are used whenever possible. Hospital pharmacists, for example, may produce intravenous drug monographs for all drugs used. For high-risk drugs such as dopamine, a standard table of administration according to the precise rate of administration required and patient's body weight will be available. Prescribers should use agreed standardized drug concentrations, and pre-printed prescriptions or stickers should be considered. Ready-made preparations must be used whenever possible to reduce the need for complicated calculations. However, despite all of these precautions, the need for dosage calculation in such patient care areas will be inevitable. Practitioners must be able to perform calculations of this nature correctly.

An independent calculation check by a second practitioner is *essential*. The selection of an appropriate administration device is also essential according to the clinical risk of the drug involved. This section begins with calculation of the rate of administration of intravenous fluids using a drip-rate controlled device. However, this type of device must *never* be used for high-risk drugs.

Calculating the rate of administration of an infusion to be given using a volumetric infusion device set in drops per minute

An *adult* volumetric-giving set administers 1 ml of infusion for every 20 drops of solution.

Care: this is different for blood-giving sets and for paediatric-giving sets. Always check the number of drops per ml for the giving-set you are using.

Example 1

You want to administer 1 l of sodium chloride 0.9% infusion over 8 hours.
Step 1: convert the volume of solution into millilitres.

1 l over 8 hours = 1000 ml over 8 hours

Step 2: calculate the volume of solution to be given per hour.

$$1000 \text{ ml over 8 hours} = \frac{1000 \text{ ml}}{8} = 125 \text{ ml per hour}$$

Step 3: calculate the volume of solution to be given per minute.

$$125 \text{ ml over 1 hour} = \frac{125}{60} = 2.08 \text{ ml per minute}$$

This could be rounded down to 2 ml per minute as this method of administration is not accurate to two decimal places.

Step 4: calculate the number of drops equivalent to this volume.
Using our chosen giving set, we must administer 20 drops to give 1 ml solution.

Therefore 2 ml = 40 drops.

Therefore, the drip controller should be set so that it administers 40 drops in one minute in order to administer 1 l of fluid over 8 hours.

Calculating the rate of administration of an infusion to be given using a high-risk infusion device set in millilitres per hour

Administration of drugs by the intravenous route is a high-risk procedure. Before administering a drug intravenously, the practitioner should check the following.

- That the situation of the patient matches the monograph available. For example, some drugs can only be given in critical care areas with appropriate close monitoring of the patient, whilst others may be given in a general ward situation.
- That the drug can be given through the available intravenous line. For example, some drugs can be given only via a central line, whilst others may also be given through a peripheral line.

- That the drug can be given through the available intravenous line in the concentration prescribed. For example, the concentration of some drug solutions varies according to whether a central or peripheral line is used.
- That the patient details correspond with the category of patient mentioned in the monograph. For example, there will be different monographs for adults, children and neonates.
- That the prescribed dose is correct for the individual patient. The monograph will normally include a statement of the correct dose to be administered according to the indication.
- That the correct diluent has been prescribed. Some drugs can only be diluted in certain diluents. For example, furosemide can only be diluted in sodium chloride 0.9% or Ringer's solution as it is incompatible with glucose solutions (BNF, 2008).
- That the correct final drug concentration has been prescribed. In some cases the final drug concentration is critical. For example, magnesium sulphate may be given in concentrations of up to 200 mg/ml (BNF, 2008).
- That the administration device is appropriate. For example, glyceryl trinitrate infusion is incompatible with polyvinyl chloride infusion containers (BNF, 2008).

Example 2

Calculate the rate of administration in millilitres per hour of dopamine infusion for a patient weighing 60 kg. You have been asked to give dopamine to go through a peripheral line at a rate of 3 micrograms/kg per minute diluted in normal saline. The patient is on a general medical ward. The recommended dilution of the infusion for peripheral administration is 800 mg dopamine in 500 ml normal saline.

Step 1: calculate the dose in micrograms/min for a 60 kg patient.

Dopamine is to be given at a rate of 3 micrograms/kg per minute. Patient weighs 60 kg.

$$3 \text{ micrograms} \times 60 \text{ kg} = 180 \text{ micrograms per minute}$$

Step 2: calculate the dose in micrograms/hour for a 60 kg patient.

$$180 \text{ micrograms/min} \times 60 \text{ mins} = 10\,800 \text{ micrograms per hour}$$

Step 3: convert the dose into milligrams per hour.

$$1 \text{ mg} = 1000 \text{ micrograms}$$
Therefore, $10\,800$ micrograms $= 10.8$ mg per hour

Step 4: check the recommended dilution of the solution for the infusion method selected and convert the calculated dose into a practical dose for administration.

> The recommended dilution of the infusion for peripheral administration is 800 mg dopamine in 500 ml normal saline. What would be the rate of administration in millilitres per hour to achieve a rate of 10.8 mg per hour?

If a solution contains 800 mg in 500 ml, how much does it contain in 1 ml?

$$\frac{1\ ml}{500\ ml} \times 800\ mg = 1.6\ mg\ in\ 1\ ml$$

Therefore, how much of the solution would contain 10.8 mg?

$$\frac{10.8\ mg}{1.6\ mg} \times 1\ ml = 6.75\ ml\ per\ hour$$

Calculating a dose for a patient on a milligrams per kilogram basis

Example 3

Calculate the dose of aminophylline to treat an adult with an acute severe asthma attack. Assume that the patient has not previously been treated with theophylline or aminophylline. The patient weighs 80 kg. You need to give a loading dose of 5 mg per kg given over 20 minutes then a maintenance dose of 500 mcg/kg per hour. The solution of aminophylline is made up as 500 mg in 500 ml.

Step 1: calculate the loading dose.

5 mg per kg × 80 kg = 400 mg over 20 min in either normal saline
or glucose 5% infusion.

Step 2: calculate the maintenance dose.

500 mcg/kg per hour in a patient weighing 80 kg = 500 × 80 mcg/h
= 40 000 mcg/h

Step 3: convert to milligrams per hour.

40 000 mcg/h = (40 000 ÷ 1000) mg/h
= 40 mg/h

Step 4: calculate the rate of administration.

The solution contains 500 mg in 500 ml, or 1 mg in 1 ml.
Therefore, the maintenance infusion should be set at 40 ml/h

Test yourself with practice calculations

1. A patient requires 1 l of glucose 5% infusion to be given over 10 hours. What is the correct rate for the drip controller in drops per minute assuming the giving set delivers 20 drops for 1 ml of solution?
2. A patient requires 500 ml sodium chloride 0.9% to be given over 4 hours. What is the correct rate for the drip controller in drops per minute assuming the giving set delivers 20 drops for 1 ml of solution?

3. Calculate the rate of administration in millilitres per hour of dobutamine infusion to be administered at a rate of 2.5 micrograms/kg per minute to a patient weighing 65 kg. The standard solution concentration recommended in your local IV monograph is dobutamine 250 mg in 500 ml sodium chloride 0.9% infusion.

4. Calculate the rate of administration in millilitres per hour of dopamine infusion to be administered at a rate of 2 micrograms/kg per minute to a patient weighing 75 kg. The standard solution concentration recommended in your local IV monograph is dopamine 800 mg in 500 ml fluid.

5. Calculate the dose of aminophylline infusion to treat an adult with an acute severe asthma attack. Assume that the patient has not previously been treated with theophylline or aminophylline. The patient weighs 85 kg. You need to prescribe a loading dose of 5 mg per kg given over 20 minutes, then a maintenance dose of 500 mcg/kg per hour. The standard solution concentration recommended in your local IV monograph is aminophylline 500 mg in 500 ml.

Answers to practice questions

Page 119

1. Try converting the following amounts:

   (a) How much is 0.5 kg in grams?
   $0.5 \times 1000 = 500$ g

   (b) How much is 62.5 mg in micrograms?
   $62.5 \times 1000 = 62\,500$ micrograms

   (c) How much is 250 micrograms in milligrams?
   $250 \div 1000 = 0.25$ mg

   (d) How much is 3500 ml in litres?
   $3500 \div 1000 = 3.5$ l

   (e) How much is 1.75 l in millilitres?
   $1.75 \times 1000 = 1750$ ml

Page 122

1. The dose of propofol to induce anaesthesia in an adult aged less than 55 years is 1.5–2.5 mg/kg. Your patient weighs 70 kg and you decide to give a dose of 1.5 mg/kg. Therefore, you require a dose of 105 mg propofol. What volume of propofol 1% injection will contain this dose?

   Step 1: work out what the percentage strength means in grams per 100 ml. Propofol 1% injection contains 1 g propofol in 100 ml. Therefore, it contains 1000 mg propofol in 100 ml, or 10 mg in 1 ml.

Step 2: calculate the volume of propofol 1% injection (10 mg in 1 ml) that will contain 105 mg.

$$\frac{\text{Dose required}}{\text{Strength available}} \times \text{volume} = \text{volume required}$$

$$\frac{105}{10} \times 1 = \text{volume required}$$

Therefore, the volume of propofol 1% injection that contains 105 mg is 10.5 ml.

2. You want to give a bolus dose of 100 mg lidocaine to a patient to control ventricular arrhythmia. The injection solution you have is lidocaine injection 2%. What volume of the injection do you need to give this dose?

Step 1: work out what the percentage strength means in grams per 100 ml. Lidocaine 2% injection contains 2 g lidocaine in 100 ml. Therefore it contains 2000 mg lidocaine in 100 ml, or 20 mg in 1 ml.

Step 2: calculate the volume of lidocaine 2% injection (20 mg in 1 ml) that will contain 100 mg:

$$\frac{\text{Dose required}}{\text{Strength available}} \times \text{volume} = \text{volume required}$$

$$\frac{100}{20} \times 1 = \text{volume required}$$

Therefore, the volume of lidocaine 2% injection that contains 100 mg is 5 ml.

3. A child aged 6 years requires a dose of propranolol IV of 20 micrograms/kg. The child weighs 20 kg and therefore the total dose needed is 400 micrograms. The propranolol injection solution contains 1 mg in 1 ml. What volume of the injection solution is required to give a 400 microgram dose?

Convert the dose into milligrams: 400 micrograms ÷ 1000 = 0.4 mg

$$\frac{\text{Dose required}}{\text{Strength available}} \times \text{volume} = \text{volume required}$$

$$\frac{0.4}{1} \times 1 = 0.4 \text{ ml}$$

Therefore, the volume of propranolol 1 mg in 1 ml that contains 400 micrograms (or 0.4 mg) is 0.4 ml.

4. A child aged 15 years requires a dose of 500 micrograms of adrenaline for acute anaphylaxis (a dose used when there is doubt as to the adequacy of the circulation). The injection solution available is adrenaline 1 in 10 000. What volume of this injection solution is required to administer this dose?

Step 1: work out what the ratio strength means.

Adrenaline 1 in 10 000 = 1 g in 10 000 ml

Step 2: convert the strength of solution to milligrams.

1 g in 10 000 ml = 1000 mg in 10 000 ml

Step 3: convert the dose into milligrams.

500 mcg ÷ 1000 = 0.5 mg

Step 4: calculate the volume of solution that will contain 0.5 mg adrenaline.

$$\frac{\text{Dose required}}{\text{Strength available}} \times \text{volume} = \text{volume required}$$

$$\frac{0.5}{1000} \times 10\,000 = 5 \text{ ml}$$

Therefore, the volume of epinephrine 1 in 10 000 that contains 500 micrograms (or 0.5 mg) is 5 ml.

Page 127

1. What is the ideal body weight of the following patients?

   (a) A man who is 185 cm tall?

   Male: Ideal body weight = (0.9 × height in centimetres) − 88 kg
   = (0.9 × 185) − 88 kg
   = 78.5 kg

   (b) A woman who is 150 cm tall?

   Female: Ideal body weight = (0.9 × height in centimetres) − 92 kg
   = (0.9 × 150) − 92 kg
   = 43 kg

2. What is the dose of co-amoxiclav suspension 125/31 for a child aged 5 years weighing 18 kg? The dose is 0.25 ml/kg repeated three times a day.

   Step 1: calculate the dose.

   Dose = Patient's weight (kg) × amount per dose (ml/kg)
   = 18 kg × 0.25 ml/kg
   = 4.5 ml

   Therefore, the dose of co-amoxiclav 125/31 in 5 ml suspension would be 4.5 ml three times a day.

3. Calculate the dose of tobramycin for an adult female to treat a severe infection to be given by slow intravenous bolus injection. The dose recommended in the BNF for a *severe* infection is 5 mg/kg daily in divided doses every 6 to 8 hours. The dose must be based on ideal body weight. The patient is 165 cm tall. Tobramycin injection contains 40 mg in 1 ml.

   Step 1: calculate the patient's ideal body weight:

   Female ideal body weight (IBW) = (0.9 × height in centimetres) − 92 kg
   = (0.9 × 165) − 92 kg
   = 56.5 kg

Step 2: calculate the total *daily* dose.

$$\text{Daily dose} = \text{Patient's IBW (kg)} \times \text{amount } per \ day \text{ (mg/kg)}$$
$$= 56.5 \text{ kg} \times 5 \text{ mg/kg}$$
$$= 282.5 \text{ mg}$$

Step 3: calculate the amount per dose.
Daily dose of 282.5 mg is to be given every 6–8 hours, therefore in either three or four divided doses.

Therefore amount per dose is $282.5 \div 3 = 94$ mg every 8 hours

or

$282.5 \div 4 = 70.6$ mg every 6 hours

Step 4: calculate the volume of tobramycin solution 40 mg in 1 ml that will contain 94 mg tobramycin.

$$\frac{\text{Dose required}}{\text{Strength available}} \times \text{volume} = \text{volume required}$$
$$\frac{94}{40} \times 1 \text{ ml} = 2.35 \text{ ml}$$

or

Step 5: calculate the volume of tobramycin solution 40 mg in 1 ml that will contain 70.6 mg tobramycin.

$$\frac{\text{Dose required}}{\text{Strength available}} \times \text{volume} = \text{volume required}$$
$$\frac{70.6}{40} \times 1 \text{ ml} = 1.76 \text{ ml}$$

Note: In practice, these volumes would probably be rounded up or down to make measurement easier. For example, 2.35 ml could be rounded up to 2.5 ml or 1.76 ml could be rounded up to 2 ml. Since the ideal body weight calculation is an estimation, this would be acceptable.

4. Calculate the dose of cyclophosphamide using the low dose intravenous regimen for an adult patient with a body surface area estimated at 1.85 m². The selected dose is 120 mg/m² once a week.

Step 1: Calculate the dose for a patient with a body surface area of 1.85 m².

$$\text{Weekly dose} = 80 \text{ mg/m}^2 \times 1.85 \text{ m}^2$$
$$= 148 \text{ mg}$$

Page 130

1. A patient requires 1 l of glucose 5% infusion to be given over 10 hours. What is the correct rate for the drip controller in drops per minute assuming the giving set delivers 20 drops for 1 ml of solution?

1 l glucose 5% over 10 hours = 1000 ml/10 = 100 ml/h

$$100 \text{ ml/h} = 100/60 \qquad = 1.67 \text{ ml/min}$$

This could be rounded up to 1.7 ml/min

20 drops = 1 ml, therefore 1.7 ml = 1.7 × 20 = 34 drops per minute.

Therefore, the drip rate controller should be set so that it administers 34 drops in 1 minute.

2. A patient requires 500 ml sodium chloride 0.9% to be given over 4 hours. What is the correct rate for the drip controller in drops per minute assuming the giving set delivers 20 drops for 1 ml of solution?

500 ml sodium chloride 0.9% over 4 hours = 500/4

$$= 125 \quad 125 \text{ ml/h}$$

$$125 \text{ ml/h} \qquad = 125/60 \qquad = 2.08 \text{ ml/min}$$

rounded down to 2 ml/min

20 drops = 1 ml, therefore 2 ml = 2 × 20 = 40 drops per minute

Therefore, the drip rate controller should be set so that it administers 40 drops in 1 minute.

3. Calculate the rate of administration in millilitres per hour of dobutamine infusion to be administered at a rate of 2.5 micrograms/kg per minute to a patient weighing 65 kg. The standard solution concentration recommended in your local IV monograph is dobutamine 250 mg in 500 ml sodium chloride 0.9% infusion.

2.5 mcg/kg per minute for a 65 kg patient = 2.5 × 65 mcg/min = 162.5 mcg/min

162.5 mcg/min = 162.5 × 60 mcg/h = 9750 mcg/h

Convert to milligrams per hour: 1000 mcg = 1 mg

Therefore: 9750 mcg/h = 9.75 mg/h

Solution contains 250 mg dobutamine in 500 ml saline, how much does it contain in 1 ml?

$$250 \text{ mg in 500 ml} = \frac{1 \text{ ml}}{500 \text{ ml}} \times 250 \text{ mg} = 0.5 \text{ mg in 1 ml}$$

What volume will contain 9.75 mg?

9.75 mg / 0.5 mg × 1 ml = 19.5 ml/h

Therefore, the pump should be set to administer 19.5 ml/h

4. Calculate the rate of administration in millilitres per hour of dopamine infusion to be administered at a rate of 2 micrograms/kg per minute to a patient weighing 75 kg. The standard solution concentration recommended in your local IV monograph is dopamine 800 mg in 500 ml fluid.

2 mcg/kg per minute in a patient weighing 75 kg = 150 mcg/min

$$150 \text{ mcg/min} \times 60 = 9000 \text{ mcg/h}$$

Convert to milligrams per hour: 1000 mcg = 1 mg

Therefore: 9000 mcg = 9 mg

Dopamine solution contains 800 mg in 500 ml, how much does it contain in 1 ml?

$$\frac{1 \text{ ml}}{500 \text{ ml}} \times 800 \text{ mg} = 1.6 \text{ mg in 1 ml}$$

$$\frac{9 \text{ mg}}{1.6 \text{ mg}} \times 1 \text{ ml} = 4.625 \text{ ml/h}$$

Therefore, the pump should be set to administer 5.63 ml/h

5. Calculate the dose of aminophylline infusion to treat an adult with an acute severe asthma attack. Assume that the patient has not previously been treated with theophylline or aminophylline. The patient weighs 85 kg. You need to prescribe a loading dose of 5 mg per kg given over 20 minutes then a maintenance dose of 500 mcg/kg per hour. The standard solution concentration recommended in your local IV monograph is aminophylline 500 mg in 500 ml.

Loading dose

5 mg per kg × 85 kg = 425 mg over 20 min

in either normal saline or glucose 5% infusion

Maintenance dose

500 mcg/kg per hour in a patient weighing 85 kg = 500 × 85 mcg/h

$$= 42\,500 \text{ mcg/h}$$

Convert to milligrams per hour: = 42.5 mg/h

The solution contains 500 mg in 500 ml, or 1 mg in 1 ml.
Therefore, the maintenance infusion should be set at 42.5 ml/h.

References

Anon. (2000). Boots pharmacist and trainee cleared of baby's manslaughter, but fined for dispensing a defective medicine. *PJ*, **264**, 390–2.

Apkon M, Leonard J, Probst L, DeLizio L, Vitale R. (2004). Design of a safer approach to intravenous drug infusions: failure mode effects analysis. *Quality and Safety in Health Care*, **13**, 265–71.

BMJ Publishing Group Ltd, Royal Pharmaceutical Society of Great Britain, RCPCH. *BNF for Children*. 2008. Oxon: Pharmaceutical Press.

British Medical Association and Royal Pharmaceutical Society of Great Britain.

(September 2007). *British National Formulary 54*. Oxon: Pharmaceutical Press.

Du Bois D, Du Bois E. (1916). A formula to estimate the approximate surface area if height and weight be known. *Archives of Internal Medicine*, **17**, 863–71.

Expert Group on Safe Medication Practices (2006). Creation of a better medication safety culture in Europe: building up safe medication practices. URL: http://www.esqh.net/Members/lnetwork/workgroup_files/Final_draft_report_safe_medication_280307.doc (accessed 26th January 2008).

Hutton M, Gardner H. (2005). Calculation skills. *Paediatric Nursing*, **17**(2), 1–17.

URL: http://www.cf.ac.uk/mathssupport/ learningresources/mathsforhealth/ pncalculationskills.pdf (accessed 27th January 2008).

Institute for Safe Medication Practices (1997). Insulin errors–abbreviations will get U in trouble. *ISMP Medication Safety Alert: Acute Care*. August 13 1997. URL: http://www.ismp.org/Newsletters/ acutecare/articles/19970813.asp (accessed 26th January 2008).

Institute for Safe Medication Practices (2000). FDA Advise-ERR: Medication errors associated with levothyroxine products. *ISMP Medication Safety Alert: Acute Care*. September 6 2000. URL: http://www.ismp.org/Newsletters/ acutecare/articles/20000906_2.asp?ptr (accessed 26th January 2008).

Institute for Safe Medication Practices (2003). Double checks for endogenous and exogenous errors. *ISMP Medication Safety Alert: Acute Care*. October 30 2003. URL: http://www.ismp.org/Newsletters/ acutecare/articles/20031030.asp (accessed 26th January 2008).

Institute for Safe Medication Practices (2007a). ISMP's List of High-Alert Medications. URL: www.ismp.org (accessed 8th January 2008).

Institute for Safe Medication Practices (2007b). Fatal 1000-fold overdoses can occur, particularly in neonates, by transposing mcg and mg. *ISMP Medication Safety Alert: Acute Care*. September 6, 2007. URL: http://www. ismp.org/newsletters/acutecare/archives/ Sep07.asp (accessed 26th January 2008).

Institute for Safe Medication Practices (2008). ISMP's List of Error-prone Abbreviations, Symbols and Dose Designations. URL: http://www.ismp.org/ Tools/errorproneabbreviations.pdf (accessed 26th January 2008).

Jones PR, Wilkinson S, Davies PS. (1985). A revision of body surface area estimations. *European Journal of Applied Physiology and Occupational Physiology*, **53**(4), 376–9.

Kohn LT, Corrigan JM, Donaldson MS. (eds). (2000). To Err is Human: Building a Safer Health System. Institute of Medicine. *Committee on Quality of Health Care in America*. Washington, DC: National Academy Press.

Lesar S. (1998). Errors in the use of medication dosage equations. *Archives of Pediatrics and Adolescent Medicine*, **152**(4), 340–4.

MacLean F, Macintyre J, McDade J, Moyes D. (2003). Dose banding of chemotherapy in the Edinburgh Cancer Centre. *Pharmaceutical Journal*, **270**, 691–3.

National Patient Safety Agency (2007a). *Safety in Doses: Medication Safety Incidents in the NHS*. 4th report from the Patient Safety observatory. PSO/4. London.

National Patient Safety Agency (2007b). *Patient Safety Alert 20: Promoting Safer Use of Injectable Medicines*. National Patient Safety Agency. London.

Nursing and Midwifery Council (2004). Standards of proficiency for pre-registration nursing education. URL: http://www.nmc-uk.org/aFrameDisplay. aspx?DocumentID (accessed 9th January 2008).

Nursing and Midwifery Council (2006). Standards of proficiency for nurse and midwife prescribers. URL: http://www. nmc-uk.org/aArticle.aspx?ArticleID (accessed 9th January 2008).

Reed MJ, Fothergill J. (2007). The Livingston Paediatric Dose Calculator. *Emergency Medicine Journal*, **24**, 567–8.

Rolfe, Harper NJN. (1995). Ability of hospital doctors to calculate drug doses. *British Medical Journal*, **310**, 1173–4.

RPSGB (2007–08). Examination guidance notes for the registration examination of the Royal Pharmaceutical Society. URL: http://www.rpsgb.org/pdfs/ preregexamguid.pdf (accessed 5th January 2008).

Sabin M. (2003). Competence in Practice-Based Calculation: Issues for Nursing Education. *Occasional paper number 3.* Learning and Teaching Support Network. London. URL http://www.health. heacademy.ac.uk/publications/ occasionalpaper/occasionalpaper03.pdf (accessed 5th January 2008).

Sandwell M, Carson P. (2005). Developing numeracy in child branch students. *Paediatric Nursing*, **17**(9). URL: http:// www.nursing-standard.co.uk/ paediatricnursing/V17/n9/p2426full.asp (accessed 9th January 2008).

Scrimshire JA. (1989). Safe use of lignocaine. *British Medical Journal*, **298**, 1494.

Smith J. (2004). *Building a Safer NHS for Patients: Improving Medication Safety.* London: Department of Health.

Walton R, Dovey S, Harvey E, Freemantle N. (1999). Computer support for determining drug dose: systematic review and meta-analysis. *British Medical Journal*, **318**, 984–90.

Wang Y, Moss J, Thisted R. (1992). Predictors of body surface area. *Journal of Clinical Anesthesia*, **4**(1), 4–10

Weatherup N. (20th September 2007). Amendments to the Livingston Paediatric Dose Calculator (Letter). URL: http:// emj.bmj.com/cgi/eletters/24/8/567 (accessed 26th January 2008).

Wheeler DW, Remoundos DD, Whittlestone KD *et al.* (2004). Doctors' confusion over ratios and percentages in drug solutions: the case for standard labelling. *J R Soc Med*, **97**, 380–3.

Wheeler DW, Whittlestone KD, Salvador R *et al.* (2006). Influence of improved teaching on medical students' acquisition and retention of drug administration skills. *British Journal of Anaesthesia*, **96**(1), 48–52.

Wheeler DW, Wheeler SJ, Ringrose TR. (2007). Factors influencing doctors' ability to calculate drug doses correctly. *International Journal of Clinical Practice*, **61**(2), 189–94.

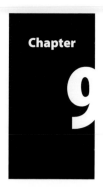

Chapter

9 Controlled Drugs and patient safety

Roger Knaggs

Patient safety is recognized increasingly as a high priority for all healthcare organizations. Managing medicines safely is central to improving patient safety. Moreover, there is increasing understanding of the frequency and causes of medication incidents, and hence systems may be developed to minimize risks associated with specific classes of drugs. No part of the system is immune to failure and in order to prevent incidents from occurring all stages of the prescribing, storage, dispensing and administration processes must be challenged. Over recent years there has been increasing interest in trying to understand the classes of medicine implicated most frequently and the settings in which these occur in order to reduce the number of medication incidents.

Opioid analgesics are frequently involved in serious medication errors (Smith, 2004) and are frequently implicated in serious errors to the NHS Litigation Authority, the Medical Defence Union and the dispensing error analysis scheme. Morphine is one of the most frequently involved drugs in medication errors in other countries too, including the United States and Sweden. In the National Patient Safety Agency (NPSA) report 'Safety in doses: medication safety incidents in the NHS' (NPSA, 2007) published in July 2007, opioids were highlighted as being most commonly implicated in medication incidents resulting in severe harm or patient death (see Table 9.1).

Opioids are widely used, in both primary and secondary care, for the management of moderate to severe pain. They are formulated to be administered by a wide range of different routes including by mouth or rectum, by the transdermal and parenteral routes, and as epidural injections and infusions. In addition, a wide range of opioid products are available and these have different potencies and release characteristics. This is worsened by the fact that opioids have a relatively narrow therapeutic margin with a fine line between providing adequate analgesia and producing side effects and toxicity. In overdose respiratory depression and hypotension may lead to patient death. However, Controlled Drugs are not just opioids. Before considering the types of incidents involving opioids and specific initiatives to improve patient safety, it is worth discussing the current legal framework relating to Controlled Drugs.

Relevant legislation

The Misuse of Drugs Act 1971 provides the legislative control over 'dangerous or otherwise harmful drugs', otherwise referred to as Controlled Drugs, the primary purpose being to prevent the misuse of Controlled Drugs. Under the Act, the possession, supply and manufacture, import and export of Controlled Drugs is prohibited excepted as allowed by the Home Office. Use of Controlled Drugs in medicine is permitted under Misuse Use of Drugs Regulations 2001 and amendments.

Medication Safety: An Essential Guide, ed. Molly Courtenay and Matt Griffiths. Published by Cambridge University Press. © M. Courtenay and M. Griffiths 2009.

Table 9.1. Medication incidents by therapeutic class, for incidents confirmed as resulting in severe harm or death

Therapeutic group	Confirmed degree of harm		Total (% of total)
	Severe harm	Death	
Opioids	5	7	12 (13%)
Anticoagulants	8	2	10 (10.9%)
Anaesthetics	3	2	5 (5.4%)
Insulin	6	2	8 (8.7%)
Antibiotics	2	3	5 (5.4%)
Chemotherapy	0	4	4 (4.3%)
Infusion fluids	1	2	3 (3.3%)
Antipsychotics	2	0	2 (2.2%)
Other	27	16	43 (46.7%)

From: Medication incidents successfully imported into NRLS database between January 2005 and June 2006 Safety in doses: medication safety incidents in the NHS (NPSA, 2007).

Table 9.2. Schedules of Controlled Drugs according to the Misuse of Drugs Regulations 2001

	Examples	Notes
Schedule 1	Hallucinogenic drugs (e.g. LSD); Ecstasy type substances; Cannabis	Little therapeutic value; Production, possession and supply limited; Home Office licence required
Schedule 2	Opioids (e.g. morphine, diamorphine, fentanyl); Major stimulants (e.g. amphetamines)	Prescription requirements; Register entries required; Safe storage required
Schedule 3	Minor stimulant drugs (e.g. benzphetamine); Buprenorphine; Midazolam, temazepam; Phenobarbitone	Prescription requirements (with exceptions); Register entries required (with exceptions); Safe storage required (with exceptions)
Schedule 4	Benzodiazepines (e.g. diazepam); Anabolic and androgenic steroids	No prescription requirements; No register entries required
Schedule 5	Preparations containing certain Controlled Drugs (e.g. codeine, morphine), which are exempt from full control	No prescription requirements; No register entries required

The classification of drugs according to the Misuse of Drugs Act is of no practical importance to practitioners as this largely relates to unlawful possession and supply of Controlled Drugs. Of more relevance is the classification of Controlled Drugs into five Schedules (Schedules 1–5) according to the Misuse of Drugs Regulations. The level of control associated with each schedule is different. For further information about the current legal requirements it is recommended to consult either '*Medicines, Ethics and Practice*' published by the Royal Pharmaceutical Society of Great Britain or the Home Office. Examples of the types of drugs that are subject to control under the Misuse of Drugs Regulations are in Table 9.2.

The Shipman Inquiry

The Shipman Inquiry was set up on 31st January 2001 after the conviction of Dr Harold Shipman, a primary care physician from Manchester, UK, who was found guilty of murdering 15 of his patients, although it has since become clear that he was responsible for at least 215 deaths. The Shipman Inquiry was chaired by Dame Janet Smith (now Lady Justice Smith) and was required to investigate the role of organizations involved in investigating Dr Shipman's actions and to recommend steps that should be taken to protect patients in the future, ensuring accountability for the use of Controlled Drugs, avoiding diversion to improper use and detecting diversion if improper use occurs.

The fourth report of the Shipman Inquiry was published on 14th July 2004 and focussed on the methods used by Shipman to divert large quantities of Controlled Drugs and the reasons it was possible for him to do this for so long without being detected. The Government's response to this report (*Safer Management of Controlled Drugs*) was published in December 2004. Although the Fourth Report of the Shipman Inquiry was primarily concerned with the misappropriation of Controlled Drugs in a community setting, the legislative changes and guidance is applicable to all NHS organizations (PCTs, NHS Trusts, and Foundation Trusts), independent hospitals and care homes.

The legislative changes following the Shipman Inquiry were the first major changes since the Misuse of Drugs Act in 1971 and have been introduced over the last few years.

- All healthcare organizations were required to appoint an 'Accountable Officer' with responsibility for ensuring safe and effective use and management of Controlled Drugs.

   The Accountable Officer is responsible for all aspects of the safe and secure management of Controlled Drugs within their organization. Specifically, the Accountable Officer is required to ensure that safe systems are in place for the management and use of Controlled Drugs and for reviewing and monitoring these systems. The Accountable Officer must also ensure that declarations and self-assessments are undertaken and clear systems for logging and investigating concerns about Controlled Drugs are in place.

- Formal inspections of providers of both healthcare organizations and social care giving authority to inspectors from the Healthcare Commission, the Commission for Social Care Inspection and the Royal Pharmaceutical Society of Great Britain.

   Accountable Officers for primary care trusts were given authority to inspect general practices and other contracted primary care providers.

- The sharing of information.

   There was a legal duty of collaboration between providers, enforcement agencies, regulatory bodies and police. Accountable Officers from primary care trusts were responsible for establishing local intelligence networks whereby information can be disseminated in a timely fashion.

Guidance from the Department of Health has recommended that prescriptions for Controlled Drugs (Schedules 2, 3 and 4) should be limited to 30 days' supply. Exceptionally, to cover a justifiable clinical need and after consideration of risks, prescriptions may be issued but the reason for the decision should be clearly documented in the patient's notes. For the most up-to-date information relating to Controlled Drugs, consult the Department of Health website (http://www.dh.gov.uk/en/Healthcare/Medicinespharmacyandindustry/Prescriptions/ControlledDrugs/index.htm) or the Home Office.

Prescribing and supply of Controlled Drugs by medical practitioners

The majority of medical practitioners are able to prescribe Controlled Drugs (excluding Schedule 1 drugs) as required by their clinical practice. There are additional prescription requirements compared with drugs that are not classified by the Misuse of Drugs Act and Misuse of Drugs Regulations. A computer generated machine-written prescription is acceptable; however, the prescriber's signature must be handwritten.

In the United Kingdom, only medical practitioners who hold a special licence issued by the Home Secretary can prescribe and administer or supply diamorphine, dipipanone or cocaine in the treatment of drug addiction. Other practitioners are required to refer any addict who requires these drugs to a treatment centre.

Prescribing and supply of Controlled Drugs by non-medical prescribers

Over the last decade there has been an increase in the number of healthcare professionals who are able to prescribe. Traditionally, this has been a role for medical personnel; however, increasingly this is being extended to include other professions. The development of non-medical prescribing was designed to give patients quicker access to medicines and improve access to services, at the same time making better use of health professionals' skills.

Supplementary prescribing

Supplementary prescribing describes 'a voluntary prescribing partnership' between an independent prescriber (who must be a doctor or dentist) and a qualified supplementary prescriber, to implement an agreed patient-specific Clinical Management Plan (CMP) with the patient's agreement.

A supplementary prescriber, who may be a nurse, pharmacist, physiotherapist, chiropodist/podiatrist, radiographer or optometrist who has undertaken an approved course, may prescribe and administer any Controlled Drug (excluding Schedule 1 Controlled Drugs) as long as it is contained within a specific CMP for that patient and there is agreement between the patient, independent prescriber and supplementary prescriber.

Independent prescribing

Independent prescribing is undertaken by a practitioner who is responsible and accountable for the assessment of patients with undiagnosed conditions and for decisions about the clinical management required, including prescribing. Currently, nurses, pharmacists and optometrists are the only non-medical prescribers able to

Table 9.3. Controlled Drugs available for Nurse Independent Prescribers

Indication	Drug	Route of administration
Palliative care	Diamorphine hydrochloride	Oral / parenteral
	Morphine hydrochloride	Rectal
	Morphine sulphate	Oral / parenteral / rectal
	Oxycodone	Oral / parenteral / rectal
	Buprenorphine	Transdermal
	Fentanyl	Transdermal
Pain relief in respect of suspected MI, or for relief of acute or severe pain after trauma including in either case post-operative pain relief	Diamorphine hydrochloride	Oral / parenteral
	Morphine hydrochloride	Rectal
	Morphine sulphate	Oral / parenteral / rectal
Treatment of initial or acute alcohol withdrawal symptoms	Chlordiazepoxide	Oral Oral
Palliative care or treatment of tonic clonic seizures	Diazepam	Oral / parenteral / rectal
	Lorazepam	Oral / parenteral
	Midazolam	Parenteral / buccal
Any indication	Dihydrocodeine tartrate	Oral
	Codeine phosphate	Oral
	Co-phenotrope	Oral

use independent prescribing, although optometrists are able to prescribe from a limited formulary for eye conditions.

Nurse Independent Prescribers are able to prescribe, supply and administer a small number of Controlled Drugs for specified medical conditions as outlined in Table 9.3.

At present, Pharmacist Independent Prescribers are unable to prescribe any Controlled Drug. This includes Schedule 5 preparations, such as codeine and dihydrocodeine tablets.

There was a Home Office consultation process regarding changing the Misuse of Drugs Regulations in 2007 to allow Pharmacist and Nurse Independent Prescribers to prescribe more Controlled Drugs; however, as yet there has been no change.

Patient Group Directions

A Patient Group Direction (PGD) is a 'written instrument for the sale, supply, and / or administration of named medicines in an identified clinical situation'. It applies to groups of patients who may not be individually identified before presenting for treatment. PGDs were developed to allow the supply of medicines to a patient with a pre-identified clinical condition without necessarily being seen by a prescriber (see NPC guide 2004). Hence patients may present directly to healthcare professionals, and the healthcare professional working within the scope of the PGD is responsible for ensuring the patient meets the criteria set out in the PGD. A PGD is not intended for long-term management of a clinical condition, as this is best achieved by prescribing for an individual patient on a one-to-one basis. PGDs best fit within services where medicines use follows a predictable pattern and is less individualized.

There are only three circumstances in which a Controlled Drug may be supplied using a PGD at present. These are as follows:

- A registered nurse may supply or administer diamorphine under a PGD for the treatment of cardiac pain to a patient admitted to a coronary care unit or emergency department of a hospital;
- A registered nurse or pharmacist may supply or administer any Schedule 5 CD (e.g. oral codeine) in accordance with a valid PGD;
- A registered nurse or pharmacist may supply Part 1 Schedule 4 CD any steroids or midazolam in accordance with a valid PGD provided that it is not a drug for parenteral administration for the treatment of addiction.
- Midazolam is the only Schedule 3 CD that can be included in a PGD.

    As with the list of Controlled Drugs for non-medical prescribers, the list of Controlled Drugs that can be included in a PGD and the circumstances in which they can be supplied or administered is currently being reviewed and may be extended.

Good practice in the management of Controlled Drugs

There are two documents that are worthy of note and summarize the current legislative position and good practice relating to the use of Controlled Drugs in primary care (National Prescribing Centre, 2007) and secondary care (Department of Health, 2007). In addition to prescribing, dispensing and administration, the guide to the use of Controlled Drugs in primary care covers issues such as nurses working in the community, care homes, out of hours services and transportation. The legal position in relation to each topic is stated, together with what is considered good practice. In secondary care, issues such as use and storage of Controlled Drugs on wards and departments, and use in operating theatres and pharmacy departments are considered. Both documents should be considered essential sources for best practice relating to Controlled Drugs.

Healthcare Commission annual report on Controlled Drugs 2007

Under the legislative changes following the Shipman Inquiry described above, the Healthcare Commission (now the Care Quality Commission) was given increased responsibility for scrutiny of the new arrangements and published their first annual report in August 2008, covering the period 1st January 2007 to 31st December 2007, on the governance of these new requirements (Healthcare Commission, 2008).

The report produced 13 recommendations, many relating to the function of the local intelligence network. Interestingly, the report highlighted potential documentation issues when a person lives in a residential home. The Care Homes Regulations 2001 require the home to keep a record of all medicines kept for the service user, and the date on which they were administered. Although nurses were completing NHS documentation relating to administration, sometimes the care home records had not been completed.

Building a Safer NHS: Improving Medication Safety 2004

In 2000, the Chief Medical Officer published a report entitled 'An Organisation with a Memory' (Donaldson et al., 2000) that highlighted the magnitude of potentially avoidable events that had resulted in unintended harm to patients and that there had been little systematic learning from adverse events and service failure previously. One aim of the report was to try and reduce the number of serious errors in prescribed drugs by 40%. The government's response to this report included the formation of the National Patient Safety Agency to implement a new national system for learning from error and adverse events and promote patient safety. Later, 'Building a Safer NHS: Improving Medication Safety' was published by The Chief Pharmaceutical Officer (Smith, 2004). This report described the frequency and possible causes of medication errors and highlighted drugs, patient populations and clinical settings that carry particular risks. Drugs that were highlighted in this report included oral anticoagulants, chemotherapy, intravenous infusions, methotrexate, potassium, drugs in anaesthesia and opioid analgesics.

Recommendations around the use of opioids included the following:

- NHS organizations should have local guidelines in place to ensure safe prescribing, dispensing and administration and monitoring of strong analgesics. Where appropriate, this may include pre-printed prescriptions;
- The range of products available for administration should be limited to minimize the risk of confusion. High-strength ampoules of opiates should not be held routinely in general ward areas or by community practitioners;
- Medical, nursing and pharmacy staff should be familiar with the range of oral morphine products available and the usual frequencies in which they are prescribed and administered;
- Patients receiving injectable or high-dose oral opiates should be monitored carefully. The opiate antagonist, naloxone, should be available and staff trained in its use. It should be prescribed in advance or the subject of a Patient Group Direction to allow its administration in an emergency;
- All acute hospitals should have a multidisciplinary pain team to advise on good practice, establish safe systems and train other staff in the safe use of strong analgesics;
- Oral sustained release opiates are a particular source of error and care should be taken to avoid any possible ambiguity when prescribing these drugs. Including the brand name on the prescription and dispensing label will aid in the identification of the correct formulation to be dispensed or administered;
- All dose calculations and drug administration of strong analgesics on hospital wards should be double checked;
- Prescriptions dispensed for individual patients to take at home should be double checked for accuracy; and
- Ideally, doses of opiates for administration to neonates and small children should be prepared centrally in the pharmacy or supplied in small dose units.

NPSA *Patient Safety Observatory 4* 2007

'Safety in Doses: Medication Safety Incidents in the NHS' (NPSA, 2007) reported 92 medication incidents in total over an 18-month period that resulted in severe harm or death to a patient. From these, the two therapeutic groups most commonly implicated were opioids and anticoagulants (see Table 9.1 earlier). Nine of the 12 reports of severe harm or death due to opioids were associated with overdose. The report emphasizes 'It is imperative that every patient receives the appropriate dose of opioid and that patients receiving opioids are monitored regularly.' Examples of the types of incident reported to the National Learning and Reporting System are provided. Despite the warnings provided and various patient safety initiatives, it appears that opioids are still associated with significant risks that cause patient harm.

NPSA *Patient Safety Alert 12* Ensuring safer practice with high dose ampoules of diamorphine and morphine (May 2006)

Following a number of reports of death and serious harm to patients due to the administration of high dose diamorphine or morphine injections to patients who had previously not received opioids, the NPSA published recommendations to improve safe practice with these medicines.

Significant risks with injectable opioid medicines had been identified and the Patient Safety Alert attempted to address these and other related issues. Prior to this time, packaging and labelling for ampoules of different strengths was very similar and ampoules containing 5 mg, 10 mg, 30 mg and 60 mg diamorphine had almost identical appearances. It was extremely common practice to store higher strength (30 mg and above) alongside lower strength products in clinical areas, both in primary and secondary care settings. Insufficient training and understanding on the part of healthcare staff of the risks when prescribing, dispensing and administering higher doses of diamorphine and morphine injections had also been highlighted.

Patient Safety Alert 12 required NHS organizations to:

- risk assess and have procedures for safely prescribing, labelling, supplying, preparing and administering diamorphine and morphine injections;
- review therapeutic guidelines for the use of diamorphine and morphine injectable products for patients requiring acute care, including post-administration observation of patients who have not previously received doses of opiates;
- update information concerning the safe use of diamorphine and morphine injectable products as part of an ongoing programme of training for healthcare staff on medication practice; and
- ensure that naloxone injection is available in all clinical locations where diamorphine and morphine injections are stored or administered.

Since the publication of this *Patient Safety Alert*, there have been significant changes to the packaging of injectable opioid products, ensuring that there is greater differentiation between different strengths of morphine and diamorphine. High-strength products also contain an additional warning label as a reminder such as 'Warning: High strength product'.

NPSA *Patient Safety Alert 21* Safer practice with epidural injections and infusions (March 2007)

Epidural analgesia involves the administration of local anaesthetic agents (bupivacaine, for example) and/or opioids, predominantly diamorphine or fentanyl, very close to the spinal column. This method of drug delivery reduces the incidence of some complications of major surgery, including chest injections and venous thromboembolism. Following the development of acute pain services in almost all hospitals in the United

Table 9.4. Types of epidural incidents reported to the NRLS from 1st January 2005 to 31st May 2006

Type of Incident	Number
Wrong route (epidural administered by IM / IV routes)	8
Wrong route (IV medicine administered by epidural route)	12
Wrong epidural drug	36
Wrong epidural dose	23
Error with other drug therapy when receiving epidural therapy	81
Documentation error	49
Error with programming or operating the infusion pump	31
Omitted epidural therapy	21
Supply error	20
Expired epidural infusion used	13
Incorrect storage of epidural medicine	8
Other	44

From NPSA *Safety Alert 21* Safer practice with epidural injections and infusions.

Kingdom, it has become increasingly common for epidural analgesia to be administered to patients on general surgical wards and not solely in critical care areas.

Between 2000 and 2004 there were at least three patient deaths reported in the lay media following the administration of epidural bupivacaine infusions by the intravenous route, highlighting the risks associated with epidural administration. Reviewing reports made to the NPSA between January 2005 and May 2006, there were 346 incidents that had been related to epidural injections and infusions (see Table 9.4 for the types of incident report). Although most resulted in no or little harm to the patient, a number of risks were highlighted, including how the medicines were stored, labelled and administered.

The recommendations relate to use for acute pain management for both children and adults including epidural injections, infusions, administering bolus doses (top-ups) and patient-controlled epidural analgesia, but were not intended for use in the specialist settings of palliative care and persistent non-cancer pain. This guidance was intended to complement consensus guidance produced by a group of European professional groups (Royal College of Anaesthetists *et al.*, 2004).

Patient Safety Alert 21 required organizations in the NHS and independent sector to take the following steps to minimize risk when administering epidural injections and infusions:

- clearly label infusion bags and syringes for epidural therapy with '**For Epidural Use Only**'. Make judicious use of colour and design to differentiate these products from those for administration by intravenous and other routes;
- minimize the likelihood of confusion between different types and strengths of epidural injections and infusions by
    rationalizing the range of products available;
    maximizing the use of ready to administer infusions to help reduce the need for complex calculations and preparations;

- reduce the risk of the wrong medicine being selected by storing epidural infusions in separate cupboards from those holding intravenous and other types of infusions;
- use clearly labelled epidural administration sets and catheters that distinguish them from those for intravenous and other routes;
- use infusion and syringe devices for epidural infusions that are easily distinguishable from those used for other routes; and
- ensure all staff involved in epidural therapy have received adequate training and have necessary work competences to undertake their duties safely.

NPSA *Rapid Response Report 05* Reducing dosing errors with opioid medicines (July 2008)

Despite *Patient Safety Alert 12*, which related to injectable opioid medicines, there continued to be reported errors in which patients received unsafe doses of opioid medicines, where the dose or formulation was incorrect, compared with previous doses. As shown in Table 9.5, there is a wide range of opioid drugs and different formulations available. In addition, patient response to opioids varies markedly and this is partly dependent on previous doses taken. Commonly, errors occur around the time of initiation of opioid therapy. Errors can also happen during dose conversion from one opioid to another or with an unintended dose increase for a patient already taking an opioid.

Rapid Response Report 05 required organizations in the NHS and independent sector to ensure: that when opioid medicines are prescribed, dispensed or administered, in anything other than acute emergencies, the healthcare practitioner concerned, or their clinical supervisor, should:

- confirm any recent opioid dose, formulation, frequency of administration and any other analgesic medicines prescribed for the patient;

Table 9.5. Opioid medicines involved in patient safety incidents

Drug	Number	Percent
Morphine	2441	55
Fentanyl	544	12
Oxycodone	520	12
Methadone	371	8
Diamorphine	293	7
Buprenorphine	135	3
Pethidine	86	2
Hydromorphone	8	0
Meptazinol	6	0
Dipipanone	3	0

From NPSA Rapid Response Report 05. Reducing dosing errors with opioid medicines.

- ensure where a dose increase is intended, that the calculated dose is safe for the patient (e.g. for oral morphine or oxycodone in adult patients, not *normally* more than 50% higher than the previous dose; and
- ensure they are familiar with the following characteristics of that medicine and formulation: usual starting dose, frequency of administration, standard dosing increments, symptoms of overdose and common side effects.

Clearly, the key to successful implementation of this Report is education of all staff involved in the prescribing, dispensing and administration of opioid medicines. This should start by providing a good understanding of basic pharmacology in undergraduate curricula but must be continued in the workplace.

NPSA Rapid Response Report 11 Reducing risk of overdose with midazolam injection in adults (December 2008)

Midazolam is a benzodiazepine used for procedural sedation, as pre-medication prior to surgery and in palliative care. Midazolam is currently available as ampoules containing 10 mg in 2 ml and 10 mg in 5 ml, both of which exceed the dose required for most patients and this is considered to be a contributing factor in the risk of using midazolam injections. This *Rapid Response Report* advocates the use of smaller ampoules in most clinical areas.

All organizations where midazolam is used for adult conscious sedation are required to check the following:

- ensure that the storage and use of high-strength midazolam (5 mg/ml in 2 ml and 10 ml ampoules; or 2 mg/ml in 5 ml ampoules) is restricted to general anaesthesia, intensive care, palliative medicine and clinical areas/situations where its use has been formally risk assessed, for example, where syringe drivers are used;
- ensure that, in other clinical areas, storage and the use of high-strength midazolam is replaced with low-strength midazolam (1 mg/ml in 2 ml or 5 ml ampoules);
- review therapeutic protocols to ensure that guidance on the use of midazolam is clear and the risks, particularly for the elderly or frail, are fully assessed;
- ensure all heathcare professionals involved directly or participating in sedation techniques have the necessary knowledge, skills and competences required;
- ensure stocks of flumazenil are available where midazolam is used and that the use of flumazenil is regularly audited as a marker of excessive dosing of midazolam; and
- ensure that sedation is covered by organizational policy and that the overall responsibility is assigned to a senior clinician, who, in most cases, will be an anaesthetist.

Opioids in cancer pain and palliative care

In 1986, the World Health Organization produced guidance on the use opioids in the management of cancer pain and a stepwise approach was suggested. This was largely aimed as a public health tool to try and increase the availability of opioids

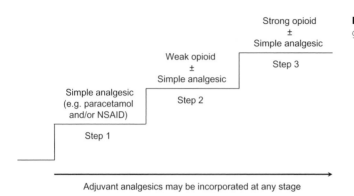

Figure 9.1. WHO analgesic ladder.

Adjuvant analgesics may be incorporated at any stage

NSAID – Non-steroidal anti-inflammatory drug

in developing countries. Principles governing use are that, where possible, analgesics should be used:

- 'By the mouth' – i.e. orally
- 'By the clock' – i.e. regularly
- 'By the ladder' (see Fig. 9.1)

Despite these principles being used for over two decades, the prevalence of unrelieved cancer pain is still extremely high and there is still widespread 'opioidphobia' with under-utilization of adjuvant analgesics.

For specific information regarding individual products and conversion between different drugs, referral to appropriate reference sources, such as the *British National Formulary* or the *Palliative Care Formulary*, is recommended.

Opioids in persistent non-cancer pain

Increasingly, strong opioids are being used in settings other than acute pain and palliative care. There is short-term evidence that some types of chronic musculoskeletal and neuropathic pains will respond to strong opioid analgesics, providing analgesia and improved quality of life. However, in addition to concerns of tolerance, dependence and addiction, long-term immunological and hormonal side effects are becoming apparent that may restrict use. The challenges facing healthcare professionals that recommend or prescribe strong opioids for non-cancer pain require identifying patients that may respond to opioids, managing medication related side effects and alleviating suffering without significantly increasing illicit use or addiction. The British Pain Society has provided recommendations and a useful patient information leaflet for the use of opioids in persistent non-cancer pain (British Pain Society, 2004).

One particular drug worthy of mention is fentanyl. When administered by the transdermal route, it is used for the treatment of severe cancer and non-cancer pain. It is available in patches that deliver 12.5, 25, 50, 75 and 100 micrograms per hour. These figures may seem rather small. However, it must be remembered that fentanyl is an extremely potent and lipophilic opioid. It may take up to 24 hours to achieve therapeutic plasma concentrations on initial application and, conversely, it may take a similar length of time for plasma concentrations to fall on removal of a patch. A patch delivering 25 micrograms per hour is equivalent to approximately 90 mg morphine sulphate orally each day.

Prescribing and dispensing opioids including brand name

When only one brand of a medicine is available, both patients and professionals alike know the product that will be dispensed by a community pharmacist. However, a problem arises when a prescription is written generically and there is more than one product available. If a prescription is written for modified release morphine sulphate tablets, it is not clear if Morpghesic® SR, MST Continus®, MXL® or Zomorph® is intended for the patient. In this circumstance the community pharmacist may dispense either the leading brand or a 'branded generic' product available from generic pharmaceutical manufacturing companies and the prescriber does not know the product that will be dispensed unless a brand name is specified on the prescription. If a prescriber does not know the brand, then a patient may be confused if she receives a medicine that she is unfamiliar with and this may compromise patient safety.

Consider the range of oral morphine formulations available. There are seven immediate release formulations, with five strengths ranging from 10 mg to 100 mg. Contrast that with 26 modified release preparations with strengths 5 mg to 200 mg. Those of us working in pain medicine know that immediate release formulations are normally taken every 4 to 6 hours and that modified release formulations are usually taken either every 12 hours or every 24 hours. There may be very good clinical reasons why one product is preferred over another (e.g. once daily formulation or mixed with semi-solid foods, where swallowing is difficult). However, if a prescription is written only using a generic name, the wrong product may be dispensed or administered.

Some products have similar sounding names or spellings, which also may be a source of confusion in prescribing, dispensing and administration. The Chief Pharmaceutical Officer highlighted this as an error in a report 'Building a Safer NHS for Patients: Improving Medication Safety' in 2004 (Smith, 2004). Examples included fatalities because of confusion between MST® and Severdol®. More recently, the fourth report of the NPSA Patient Safety Observatory noted that opioids were responsible for more cases of severe harm to the patient or death than any other class of drug, and that modified release formulations were implicated in incidents, particularly in relation to picking the wrong formulation of the same medicine. The Chief Pharmaceutical Officer suggested that, to minimize the chance of errors in prescribing, dispensing and administration, the brand (proprietary) name and generic (drug) name should be included on both the prescription and dispensing label.

This is not just a problem for modified release morphine formulations. After having witnessed the potential for confusion with different transdermal preparations, Andrew Dickman, a palliative care pharmacist from Liverpool, suggested that brand prescribing should be adopted for all strong opioids. In February 2006, the Royal Pharmaceutical Society's Practice Committee endorsed this practice for both modified release morphine and transdermal fentanyl preparations, although it would be logical to extend it to all oral modified release opioid formulations, whether for oral or transdermal delivery. This position was endorsed by the Council of the British Pain Society. However, prior to this, the RPSGB Council had reviewed its position stating 'that there is no compelling evidence to show switching brands of modified release morphine preparation with the same release profile affects pain control. Also, there is no evidence of a difference in the rate of delivery between brands of fentanyl patches when used in accordance with the product licence.'

Despite this, a recent palliativedrugs.com survey (palliativedrugs.com, 2007) suggested that 78% of respondents had patients who had confused immediate release opioid formulations with modified release opioid formulations, with 41% also reporting pharmacists dispensing the wrong product. Almost half of all clinicians (43%) thought these errors had led to a serious undesirable effect. Analysing 47 more detailed responses, the majority indicated loss of pain control and/or opioid toxicity as the most serious undesirable effect; however, five in-patient admissions were reported and two responses suggested more serious consequences (fall leading to fracture and head trauma).

The patient's preference

If the preparation looks different every time it is dispensed, it is not surprising that a patient becomes confused. As the majority of patients are taking other medicines for co-morbidities, changes – particularly in brand name and outer packaging – may lead to the assumption that a new medicine is intended. Patients may also prefer one preparation over another because of its shape, size, taste, colour or the ease with which the packaging opens.

Where possible, the brand of modified release opioid should not be changed unintentionally. If the brand needs to be changed, then the patient and the patient's carers must understand and accept the need for change. It is the responsibility of all healthcare professionals to ensure that patients take their medicines correctly by appropriate questioning and suitable patient counselling.

Summary

Controlled Drugs are subject to the legislation contained in the Misuse of Drugs Act 1971 and Regulations that are made under the Act. These requirements are greater than for other medicines, partly to minimize abuse and addiction potential. For many years there had been relatively few legislative changes relating to Controlled Drugs; however, the Shipman Inquiry recommended major changes, particularly in strengthening of the governance arrangements. The development of additional methods of prescribing by non-medical healthcare practitioners and supply using Patient Group Directions has also required legislative changes to accommodate these extended roles.

As well as being subject to specific legislation, Controlled Drugs are some of the most potent medicines to cause respiratory depression and potentially are lethal if administered in too large quantities. In the United Kingdom and other countries opioids have been highlighted as being associated with many medication errors and patient safety incidents. Hence there has been interest in trying to maintain the balance between encouraging safe practice with opioids and ensuring availability for the treatment of severe pain. Issues of similarities between high-strength and low-strength ampoules of morphine and diamorphine, risks associated with epidural injections and infusions, and risks associated with prescribing, dispensing and administering opioid medicines have been the subject of reports by the National Patient Safety Agency. The key message must be that, whilst Controlled Drugs are used widely, they must be treated with a great deal of respect too.

References

British Pain Society (2004). *Recommendations for the appropriate use of opioids for persistent pain.* Available at http://www.britishpainsociety.org/book_opioid_main.pdf. Accessed 28th November 2008.

Department of Health (2007). *Safer Management of Controlled Drugs. A guide to good practice in secondary care (England).* London: DH. Available at http://www.dh.gov.uk/en/Publicationsandstatistics/Publications/PublicationsPolicyAndGuidance/DH_079618. Accessed 28th November 2008.

Dickman A. (2005). Branded prescribing of strong opioids should be adopted as good practice. *Pharmaceutical Journal,* **275**, 546.

Donaldson L. (2000). *An Organisation with a Memory.* London: DH. Available at http://www.dh.gov.uk/en/Publicationsandstatistics/Publications/PublicationsPolicy AndGuidance/DH_4065083. Accessed 15th December 2008.

Healthcare Commission (2008). *Safer Management of Controlled Drugs.* Annual report 2008. Available at http://www.healthcarecommission.org.uk/_db/_documents/The_safer_management_of_controlled_drugs_Annual_report_2007.pdf. Accessed 4th December 2008.

National Patient Safety Agency (2006). *Patient Safety Alert 12 Ensuring safer practice with high dose ampoules of diamorphine and morphine.* London: NPSA. Available at http://www.npsa.nhs.uk/nrls/alerts-and-directives/notices/morphine-diamorphine/. Accessed 11th December 2008.

National Patient Safety Agency (2007). *Patient Safety Alert 21 Safer practice with epidural injections and infusions.* London: NPSA. Available at http://www.npsa.nhs.uk/nrls/alerts-and-directives/alerts/epidural-injections-and-infusions/. Accessed 11th December 2008.

National Patient Safety Agency (2007). *Safety in doses: medication safety incidents in the NHS.* London: NPSA. Available at http://www.npsa.nhs.uk/nrls/medication-zone/reviews-of-medication-incidents/. Accessed 11th December 2008.

National Patient Safety Agency (2007). *Rapid Response Report 05. Reducing dosing errors with opioid medicines.* London: NPSA. Available at http://www.npsa.nhs.uk/nrls/alerts-and-directives/rapidrr/reducing-dosing-errors-with-opioid-medicines/. Accessed 11th December 2008.

National Patient Safety Agency (2008). *Rapid Response Report 11. Reducing risk of overdose with midazolam injections in adults.* London: NPSA. Available at http://www.npsa.nhs.uk/nrls/alerts-and-directives/rapidrr/reducing-risk-of-overdose-with-midazolam-injection-in-adults/. Accessed 11th December 2008.

National Prescrbing Centre (2004). *Patient Group Directions. A practical guide and framework of competencies for all professionals using patient group directions.* Available at http://www.npc.co.uk/publications/pgd/pgd.pdf. Accessed 28th November 2008.

National Prescribing Centre (2007). *A guide to good practice in the management of controlled drugs in primary care (England).* Available at http://www.npc.co.uk/controlled_drugs/CDGuide_2ndedition_February_2007.pdf. Accessed 28th November 2008.

Palliativedrugs.com. Newsletter January / February 2007. Available at http://www.palliativedrugs.com/view-legacy-newsletter?&;nlid = 360. Accessed 11th December 2008.

Royal College of Anaesthetists, Royal College of Nursing, Association of Anaesthetists of Great Britain and Northern Ireland, British Pain Society, European Society of Regional Anaesthesia (2004). *Good practice in the management of continuous epidural analgesia in the hospital setting.* Available at http://www.rcoa.ac.uk/docs/epid-analg.pdf. Accessed 4th December 2008.

Smith J. (2004). *Building a safer NHS for patients: improving medication safety.* London: DH. Available at http://www.dh.gov.uk/en/ Publicationsandstatistics/Publications/ Publications PolicyAndGuidance/ DH_4071443. Accessed 11th December 2008.

Chapter 10

Reporting medication errors and near misses

Sheena Williamson

Medication safety incidents

Introduction

Between January 2005 and June 2006 there were 59 802 medication safety incidents reported via the National Reporting and Learning System (NRLS) in England and Wales. Medication incidents are the second most commonly reported incident next to patient accidents (NPSA, 2007).

Although there has been an increase in reporting over the last 3 years, literature suggests gross inconsistencies and substantial under-reporting from a large number of NHS organizations (NPSA, 2007). This has been borne out in a systematic review of international literature from 12 countries suggesting the average rate of under-reporting of adverse drug events is as high as 94% (Hazell & Shakir, 2006).

A significant proportion of low reporting or non-reporting has arisen from primary care organizations with only 4.9% of the total medication incidents reported to the NRLS coming from the primary care setting.

The aim of this chapter is to define what is meant by medication safety incidents and to examine where errors are likely to occur within the medication process, including a brief overview of some of the findings in the data that are pertinent to reporting medication incidents from the National Patient Safety Agency Report (2007) Safety in doses: medication safety incidents in the NHS. The main section in the chapter consists of guidance on how to report medication incidents, utilizing the recommendations from NPSA on how to improve reporting.

Terms and definitions

The National Patient Safety Agency (NPSA) has defined a patient safety incident as 'any unintended or unexpected incident which could have or did lead to harm for one or more patients' (NPSA, 2004). A wide variety of terms are used in the definition and classification of medication safety incidents and it is important to understand the differences between each of these. The model in Fig. 10. 1 demonstrates the correlation between the terms explained below.

Medication errors are broadly defined as incidents in which an error has occurred somewhere in the medication process, regardless of whether any harm occurred to the patient.

Potential Adverse Drug Events (near misses) may be identified as incidents which did not cause any harm at the time but may have had the potential to cause harm. Near misses are often under-reported and yet they provide rich data to help improve the management of systems to reduce risks and improve patient safety.

Medication Safety: An Essential Guide, ed. Molly Courtenay and Matt Griffiths. Published by Cambridge University Press. © M. Courtenay and M. Griffiths 2009.

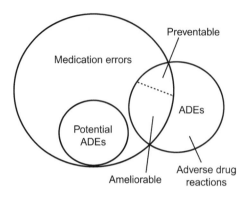

Figure 10.1. Demonstrates the correlation between medication errors, potential adverse drug events and preventable adverse drug events and non preventable adverse drug reactions (Morimoto *et al.*, 2004)

Adverse Drug Events ADEs (actual harm from medicines) are medication incidents defined as 'any undesirable experience that has happened to the patient while taking a drug but which may or may not be related to the drug' (MHRA, 2006).

Adverse drug events may be divided into two categories.

A **preventable ADE** is an injury that is the result of an error at any stage throughout the medication process.

A **non-preventable ADE** is an injury due to a medication where there is no error in the medication process. These are also referred to as **Adverse Drug Reactions (ADRs)**. The MHRA defines an ADR as 'an unwanted or harmful reaction experienced following the administration of a drug or a combination of medications, and is suspected to be related to the medication. The reaction may be a known side effect of the medication or it may be new and previously unrecognized'.

The NPSA collects data on **all types** of medication error and the MHRA collects data on adverse drug reactions via the Yellow Card system. Therefore, it is important that information is shared and data are processed between each of these organizations.

Medication errors within the medication process

The medication process is the term used to describe the process of delivering medications to patients. It consists of five stages.

Stage 1: Prescribing the medicine.

Stage 2: Dispensing the medicine.

Stage 3: Preparing the medicine for administration.

Stage 4: Administering the dose using the appropriate route and method.

Stage 5: Monitoring the effect of the medicine on the patient (NPSA, 2007).

The potential for error lies within each stage.

Stage 1: Prescribing errors

Prescribing medicines is now no longer the sole responsibility of medical staff. A number of nurses, pharmacists and optometrists have undertaken education to enable them to independently prescribe almost all the medications in the *British National Formulary*, within their scope of clinical practice. Similarly, a number of allied health professions (physiotherapists, radiologists, chiropodists/podiatrists) and optometrists, nurses and pharmacists may prescribe as supplementary prescribers, in partnership with a medical practitioner.

A prescribing error may be defined as the incorrect drug selection for a patient or errors involving wrong drug, dose, quantity, indication for use or a contraindication (Williams, 2007). Prescribing errors also include illegible handwriting, misspelling of a drug with a similar name and use of abbreviations.

Prescription errors are estimated as being between <1% and 11% of all written prescriptions (Sanders & Esmail, 2003).

Stage 2: Dispensing errors

Dispensing is carried out in a variety of settings from hospital pharmacies, community pharmacies and some rural General Practices. One common dispensing error is selection of the wrong product, usually where there are two drugs with similar proprietary names (e.g. Losec® and Lasix®), which may look similar when hand written. Other dispensing errors include wrong dose, wrong drug and wrong patient and some reports suggest typing errors in computerized labelling as a common cause of error in dispensing (Williams, 2007).

Stage 3 and 4: Administration and preparation errors

There is very little documented data around preparation and administration errors occurring in patients in the community. However, there is a reported wide variation in the rates of preparation and administration error within hospitals with rates varying between 3.5% and 49% (NPSA, 2007). The NPSA also suggest that this wide range reflects the differences in the definitions used to record medication error, together with methods of data collection.

Drug administration and preparation has been considered as an area of 'high risk' within nursing practice and the well-known six *Rights of the Medication Use Process* should be familiar to all:

- Right patient
- Right drug
- Right dose
- Right route
- Right time
- Right outcome

Many drug administration errors are errors of omission but also include failure to check patient identity, incorrect administration technique and administration of a wrong or expired drug (Williams, 2007).

The literature suggests that the medication error rate for administration of intravenous (IV) drugs may be as high as 25% and these errors have significant risk to patients (Bruce & Wong, 2001).

One of the most common types of error identified is 'deliberate violation of guidelines', for example, where practitioners have injected IV medication faster than the recommended time stated in the guidelines (Williams, 2007).

Stage 5: Errors in monitoring outcome

With an increasing elderly population, there is a subsequent rise in patients living with long-term, often complex chronic diseases. This gives rise to issues of medicines management and the need for careful monitoring of outcomes. Some patients take certain drugs, which require continuous monitoring to ensure they are taking the optimum dose for their condition at the time. Literature suggests that recommended ongoing monitoring of patients taking certain drugs is not being undertaken by healthcare professionals. The NPSA (2007) cite one study where less than one-third of patients taking diuretics were having the electrolyte levels in their blood monitored. This statement may be borne out by evidence stating diuretics as one of the medicines most commonly responsible for medicine-related admission to hospital (Pirmohamed *et al.*, 2004; Howard *et al.*, 2007).

The Nursing and Midwifery Council (NMC) has produced Standards for Medicines Management (2007), which sets standards for safe practice for supplying, administering and dispensing medicines to patients.

There are also Standards of Proficiency for Nurse and Midwife Prescribers (2006) and both these documents are available via the following link: http://www.nmc-uk.org/.

The extent of the problem

The Department of Health estimates that the annual cost of avoidable hospital admissions resulting from drug errors cost in the region of £200–400 million per annum.

Pirmohamed *et al.* (2004) carried out the largest UK study of hospital admissions data over 6 months and their findings concluded that 6.5% of all admissions were related to harm from medicines. From these findings the researchers concluded that 4.7% of all admissions were as a result of avoidable harm from medicines. The medicines most commonly responsible were aspirin, diuretics, warfarin and non-steroidal anti-inflammatory drugs. More recently, a systematic review of international literature by Howard *et al.* (2007) cited the drugs most commonly responsible for medicine-related admission were antiplatelets, diuretics, non-steroidal anti-inflammatory drugs and anticoagulants, which supports the UK figures.

The National Patient Safety Agency and The National Reporting and Learning System

England and Wales

The National Patient Safety Agency (NPSA) was set up in 2001 and one of its main functions was to develop the National Reporting and Learning System (NRLS), which primarily collects information on reported patient safety incidents from local risk management systems in England and Wales. The NRLS dataset is designed to collect reports from any single patient safety incident immediately after it occurs. From the data collected, themes and patterns in the types of incidents being reported may be identified including major systems failures, allowing development, promotion and implementation of solutions (WHO, 2005).

The data are confidential and no information is held on identities of individual staff or patients and the focus is on:

- characteristics of the patient
    - age
    - sex
    - ethnicity
- patient outcomes
- any contributory factors
- factors which may have prevented harm.

There is also an area for free text for detailed explanations if needed.

Brief summary of findings from the NRLS data

The NPSA report Safety in Doses: medication safety incidents in the NHS (2007), was based on reports to the NRLS over a period of eighteen months, between January 2005 and June 2006. Within the time period, 59 802 medication incidents were reported to the NRLS and these included 'near miss' incidents. Table 10.1 shows the ten most common types of reported patient safety incident. The figures demonstrate that medication incidents are the second most frequent type of incident reported after patient accidents.

Settings

From the NPSA report (2007), it would appear that there is substantial under-reporting by NHS organizations, particularly within primary care settings. Although most prescribing and dispensing is carried out in the community, over 80% of the medication incidents reported to the NRLS came from hospital reports with only 4.9% of medication incidents being reported from the primary care setting.

Non-NHS organizations such as those run by the local authority or the voluntary sector are not connected to the NRLS at present.

Table 10.1. The ten most common types of patient safety incident (NPSA, 2007)

Type of patient safety incident	Number	Percentage
Patient accident	278 886	38.8
Medication	59 802	8.3
Treatment, procedure	58 921	8.2
Access, admission, transfer, discharge (including missing patient)	55 710	7.8
Infrastructure (including staffing, facilities, environment)	46 122	6.4
Documentation (including records, identification)	35 533	4.9
Clinical assessment (including diagnosis, scans, tests, assessments)	31 644	4.4
Consent, communication, confidentiality	28 723	4.0
Medical device/equipment	23 389	3.3
Total	653 674	91.0

Age groups

Although the patient's age was indicated in less than half of all the reports to the NRLS during the 18-month period, it would appear from the data that children aged 0–4 years together with older adults peaking at 75–79 years are more likely to be involved in medication incidents.

Incident occurrence during stages of the medication process

Almost 60% of reported incidents in hospital settings occurred during administration and supply. In the community, 62.9% of incidents occurred during preparation or dispensing.

One-third of trusts (mainly primary care trusts) reported no medication incidents occurring over 6 months. More information would have been useful to support these findings as it is unclear as to whether one-third of trusts have had absolutely no medication incidents to report or whether there is a fundamental failure in their local reporting systems.

Types of medication error

Two main types of error were found in over half of the reported incidents: wrong dose, omitted medicines and wrong medicines. These types accounted for almost 50% of the reported errors. Others included wrong quantity, mismatch between patient and medicine, wrong/transposed/omitted medicine label, patient allergy to treatment, wrong storage and wrong/omitted/passed expiry date.

Outcome of error to patients

Outcomes of error were reported (Piramohamed *et al.*, 2004) by degree of harm to patients ranging from 'no harm', 'low, moderate or severe harm' to 'death'. From the data, it appeared that more medication incidents resulted in 'no harm' than all other incidents reported to the NRLS.

Also, there were less medication incidents resulting in 'death' than all other patient safety incidents reported. Although the proportion of reported harm is small, there is no room for complacency. Remember that these findings may also reflect under-reporting.

Scotland

Following a baseline study carried out in 2005, 'A Scottish prescription – managing the use of medicines in hospitals', there were key recommendations made to NHS Quality Improvement Scotland (NHS QIS). One of these recommendations was 'to develop a national approach to collecting data on adverse incidents, including medication incidents, to allow robust trend analysis, transferable lessons and benchmarking'.

Between 2005 and 2007, QIS led an initiative to develop a standardized approach to incident and near-miss reporting across NHS Scotland.

The Scottish Government established the Scottish Patient Safety Alliance in 2007 to guide the Scottish Patient Safety Programme and promote a systematic approach to improving the safety of patients in hospital. It brings together the NHS, the Scottish Government, professional bodies and patient representatives in a new drive to significantly reduce adverse events and improve patient safety (Audit Scotland, 2008).

Reporting patient safety incidents

What to report

Patient safety incidents to be reported are defined by the NPSA as 'any unintended or unexpected incident which could have or did lead to harm for one or more patients receiving NHS care'. The NRLS was developed by the NPSA to foster a culture of open reporting, in order to learn from adverse events.

The reports are anonymous, although it may be that the trust or Health Board may be identifiable. Names of patients and staff are removed prior to the information being stored in the database. Williams (2007) suggests there are significant increases in the reporting of medication errors where confidential 'no-fault' reporting has been implemented.

When to report

The NPSA encourages reporting of *all patient safety incidents* and includes the following in their criteria:

- incidents you have been involved in;
- incidents you have witnessed;
- incidents which caused no harm (or minimal harm);
- incidents resulting in moderate or severe harm (including death);
- prevented patient safety incidents (near misses).

The NPSA does not have the statutory power to make incident reporting mandatory. There have been suggestions that reporting ought to be mandatory in a bid to combat under-reporting, yet the literature examining the causal factors for under-reporting does not appear to support this idea in principle. In 1976, Dr Bill Inman highlighted 'seven deadly sins', which may account for low reporting rates. These sins, as summarized by Belton *et al.* (1995), ranged from 'ignorance' (uncertainty of how to report), 'diffidence' (looking foolish), 'fear' (of exposure to legal liability), 'lethargy' (too busy), 'guilt' (reluctant to admit cause of harm), 'ambition' (preference to publish findings) to 'complacency' (only safe drugs are marketed).

Conversely, an attitudinal survey of Dutch physicians (Elland *et al.*, 1999) reported the following findings:

only 26% knew which ADRs to report;

93% thought the reaction was too well known to warrant reporting;

75% thought the reaction was trivial;

72% were uncertain whether the reaction was caused by a drug;

33% did not have enough time;

36% thought reporting was too bureaucratic;

22% did not know how to report;

18% were not aware of the need to report.

From the Dutch findings, it could be argued that mandatory reporting may improve under-reporting, although it would appear that emphasis on the importance of reporting and education on pharmacovigilance is essential.

Who reports?

Any healthcare staff member may report a patient safety incident. Patients and carers may also report using a different form.

Participation in the reporting mechanism is voluntary.

How to report

Most trusts and health boards have an electronic risk management system, which has a link enabling reports to be submitted directly into the NRLS. Establishments which do not have a direct electronic link may use the electronic reporting form or 'eForm' which has been developed by the NPSA.

Individual healthcare workers may report either via their local risk management system or directly via the NPSA website.

The eForm may be accessed via the following link https://www.eforms.npsa.nhs.uk/staffeform/.

Patients and carers may also report safety incidents via the following link: https://www.eforms.npsa.nhs.uk/eformPP/step1.do.

What happens to the report?

The information provided in each report is fed into the NPSA database. Considerable learning can be gained from the data as this provides information on 'trends and patterns in patient safety' which enables solutions to be developed.

Lessons learned are disseminated through the publication of feedback such as:

- NRLS Quarterly Data Reports;
- Patient Safety Alerts.

Incident reports are not generally made available to the public, although some trusts and health boards may provide information to the public if deemed necessary.

Reporting adverse drug reactions (ADRs)

A recent study by Pirmohamed *et al.* (2004) determined that ADRs were related to 6.5% of adult hospital admissions and that in 80% of those, the ADR was the direct cause of admission. The study also found that ADRs accounted for 4% of all hospital admissions resulting in a projected annual cost to the NHS of £466 million. Further findings showed that the mortality rate of patients admitted with ADRs was over 2%.

Reporting of ADRs began in 1964 following the thalidomide tragedy. In 1958, Distaval® was advertised as being an 'outstandingly safe' medication which was 'relatively free from side-effects'. It was commonly given to women during the first 3 months of pregnancy to combat nausea and sleeplessness. Following a huge rise in the number of babies being born with deformities, Distaval® was withdrawn from sale in the UK from 1961.

As a direct result of the world-wide extent of the thalidomide tragedy, the Committee on Safety of Drugs was established in the UK in 1964 and was the world's first reporting mechanism for adverse drug reactions. In 1971, the Committee on Safety of Drugs became the Committee on Safety of Medicines (CSM) and in 2005, the committee became the Commission on Human Medicines (CHM). It is an expert committee within the Medicines and Healthcare Products Regulatory Agency (MHRA) whose duties include:

- advising Ministers on matters relating to human medicinal products;
- advising the Licensing Authority (LA), including giving advice in relation to the safety, quality and efficacy of human medicinal products;
- considering representations made in relation to the Commission's advice by an applicant or by a licence or marketing authorization holder;
- promoting the collection and investigation of information relating to adverse reactions for human medicines (except for those products that fall within the remit of ABRH or HMAC) for the purposes of enabling such advice to be given (MHRA, 2008).

How to report adverse drug reactions

The Yellow Card scheme

The Yellow Card scheme is a British initiative run by the MHRA and the CHM and it is used to gather information from anybody, health professionals and the general public, on suspected side effects or ADRs from:

- prescription medicines;
- herbal remedies;
- over-the-counter medicines;
- ADRs suspected to be caused by unlicensed medicines in cosmetic treatments.

The MHRA and its predecessor organizations have collected reports of suspected adverse drug reactions through the Yellow Card scheme for over 40 years. Since the establishment of the scheme, over 500 000 UK reports have been collected. The Yellow Card scheme acts as an early warning system for the identification of previously unrecognised reactions and enables identification of risk factors, outcomes of the ADR and other factors that may affect clinical management.

The continued success of the scheme is dependent on the vigilance of UK healthcare professionals and their willingness to report suspect ADRs. Every report can make a difference.

The MHRA and CHM also have five Yellow Card Centres whose role focuses on follow-up of reports in their areas as this has been shown to improve follow-up rates:

- Liverpool
- Cardiff
- Edinburgh
- Newcastle-upon-Tyne
- Birmingham.

Access to Yellow Cards

Paper copies of Yellow Cards may be found in copies of the *British National Formulary* (BNF), the *Nurse Prescribers' Formulary* (NPF), the *British National Formulary for Children* (BNFC), the *Monthly Index of Medical Specialties* (MIMS) and from the Association of the British Pharmaceutical Industry (ABPI) *Compendium of Data Sheets* and *Summaries of Product Characteristics*.

Electronic Yellow Cards may be accessed via the MHRA website www.yellowcard. gov.uk.

Who can report via the Yellow Card scheme?

All healthcare professionals and members of the general public may submit reports. It should be noted that patient reporting is undertaken using a different form within the MHRA web site.

What should be reported via the Yellow Card scheme?

Any suspected ADR should be reported through the Yellow Card scheme. If there is any doubt around whether a patient has indeed suffered from an ADR, it is good practice to report this anyway. It is important to remember that the cause does not need to be established beforehand.

It is essential to report all reactions for the following:

- black triangle drugs;
- reactions in children;
- all serious reactions from established drugs and vaccines including those that are:
  - fatal
  - life-threatening
  - disabling or incapacitating
  - result in prolonged hospitalization;
  - cause congenital abnormality;
  - medically significant;
  - areas of particular importance including:
    - delayed drug effect;
    - elderly patients;
    - ADRs associated with herbal remedies;
    - congenital anomalies.

Black triangle drugs

Black triangle products are new drugs and vaccines, which are being monitored more intensively in order to confirm the risk/benefit profile of the product. They are indicated in reference texts by the inverted black triangle symbol ▼.

Healthcare professionals are encouraged to report **all** suspected ADRs for black triangle drugs, regardless of the seriousness of the suspected reaction. Black triangle products are usually new drugs but black triangle status can also be applied to:

- a new combination of active substances (even though those substances have been previously licensed);
- administration via a new route of administration or drug delivery system/device;
- a significant new indication, which may alter the established risk/benefit profile of the product.

There is no standard time for a product to retain black triangle status. However, an assessment is usually made following 2 years of post-marketing experience and the black triangle symbol is not removed until the safety of the drug is well established (MHRA, 2008).

A list of black triangle products is available on the MHRA website: www.mhra.gov.uk.

Serious reactions of particular importance

All serious reactions should be reported via the Yellow Card scheme; however, there are some areas of particular importance to the MHRA and these include children, the elderly, delayed drug effects, congenital anomalies and ADRs associated with herbal medicines.

Reactions in children

It is important to remember that many medicines routinely used for children are not licensed for use in this age group. All suspected ADRs that occur in children under 18 years of age should be reported, regardless of whether the medicine is licensed for children or not. Monitoring of drug safety is essential for this age group as children are not generally exposed to medicines within clinical drug trials.

Reactions in elderly patients

The number of people over 65 years of age continues to grow. A high proportion of these patients receive medicines on a regular basis. The physiological changes that occur naturally with ageing have an impact on pharmacokinetics and pharmacodynamics related to drug therapy in these patients. The elderly are more susceptible to the therapeutic and adverse effects of drugs. Elderly patients often receive multiple numbers of medicines for their multiple disease states, which increases the risk of drug side effects and drug interactions. It is therefore important to monitor the safety of medicines in this age group.

The National Service Framework for Older People (2001) describes how to maximize the benefits of medicines and how to avoid excessive, inappropriate or inadequate consumption of medicines by older people.

Delayed drug effects

Delayed effects may be more difficult to monitor as they may not manifest until months or years after exposure to a particular drug. The MHRA request that any suspicion of such an association is reported.

Congenital anomalies

If a baby is born with an abnormality, or if a pregnancy results in a malformed aborted fetus, any suspicion of an adverse drug reaction during the pregnancy must be reported.

Herbal medicines

There is a history of herbal products being perceived as 'safe' as they are thought of as being natural products. From a safety point of view, it is worth considering these products in the same way as conventional medicines for the following reasons.

- Often they have not undergone adequate clinical trial testing.
- They may not have a product licence.
- They can cause unexpected adverse reactions and interact with other medicines – there is often little documented evidence with regard to adverse reactions and interactions (Barnes *et al.*, 2003).

What other information is needed?

There are four crucial pieces of information needed when reporting an ADR:

- **Suspected drug/drugs**
  - Name of drug
  - Route of administration
  - Daily dose
  - Dates of administration

- **Suspected reaction**
  - Suspected drug reaction (including diagnosis if appropriate)
  - Date of reaction
  - Seriousness of reaction
  - Any treatment given for the reaction

- **Patient details**
  - Sex of patient
  - Age at time of reaction
  - Patient's weight (if known)
  - Patient's initials and local identification number

- **Reporter details**
  - Full name and address

Any other information which may be relevant to the case should be reported.

Improving reporting of medication incidents

NPSA seven priority areas for action

The NPSA (2007) have challenged the NHS organizations in their report, 'Safety in doses: medication safety incidents in the NHS', over some of their findings highlighting weaknesses in current medication practice.

In order to improve patient safety, they have recommended seven priority actions for all staff to implement and have determined priorities for both individual healthcare professionals and for NHS organizations.

Increase reporting and learning from medication incidents

Recommendations to individual healthcare professionals.

- Report any medication incidents either directly to NRLS via the website or through the local risk management system.
- Ensure reporting medication incidents is included as an objective in personal development plans (PDPs).
- Use reflection and analysis of incidents to enhance your objectives for your PDP.

Recommendations for NHS organizations.

- Ensure commitment at strategic level to improving patient safety.
- Increase reporting of medication safety incidents.
- Ensure quality assurance processes are in place by engaging the senior pharmacists with chief executive, medical and nursing directors to ensure incident reports are completed and reviewed.
- Form a multidisciplinary group to carry out reviews of medication incidents, audit and initiate action to minimize risk.
- Ensure regular feedback is given to all healthcare workers.
- Produce a widely available annual report that summarizes incident reports and the learning gained from them.

Implement NPSA safe medication practice recommendations

Since 2001, the NPSA has produced guidance in safe medication practice, particularly to help minimize the risks associated with the 'high-risk' medication practices. These may be found on the NPSA website under Patient Safety Alerts http://www.npsa.nhs. uk/patientsafety/alerts-and-directives/alerts/.

Recommendations for individual healthcare professionals.

- Read and implement the guidance produced by the NPSA to help minimize risk in practice from these high-risk medications/medication practices.

Recommendations for NHS organizations.

- Monitor and audit the NPSA guidance and evaluate improvements following inclusion of the information.
- Share results of evaluations with Healthcare Commission and NHS litigation organizations.

Improve staff skills and competencies

The NPSA has developed multidisciplinary work-based competences as part of recent patient safety alerts such as anticoagulant therapy, the use of injectable medicines and paediatric infusions. These e-learning competences are designed to help healthcare professionals to acquire essential knowledge to allow them to practise safely.

Recommendations for individual healthcare professionals and NHS organizations.

- Use the e-learning packages to help develop competence in the safe use of medicines.
- Identify other competences which may be improved in the future by education and training.

Minimize dosing errors

From the NPSA report (2007) it would appear that dosing errors are the most frequently reported medication incident, with older adults and children being more commonly involved.

Recommendations for individual healthcare professionals.

- Make full use of all accessible, essential information (national and local medicines information services and therapeutic protocols) when prescribing, dispensing, preparing, administrating or monitoring medicines.
- *Always* undertake the required safety checks on dosages.
- If drug calculations are necessary, always have another member of staff calculate the dose independently from you.
- Ensure all clinical monitoring and dosage adjustments are in place as and when required.
- During prescribing, dispensing or administering medicines, ensure awareness of previous doses and any changes to patient's condition that may result in an alteration to the dose of medicine.

Recommendations for NHS organizations.

- Dosing errors must be audited and analysed to identify common local risks.
- Ensure all appropriate staff have access to essential information to enable them to prescribe, dispense, prepare, administer and monitor safely.
- Review local and national policies to ensure they provide accurate guidance to minimize risk.
- Ensure staff have access to (where available) calculation charts, software, syringe drivers and ready-to-use products to avoid complex dose calculations.

Ensure medicines are not omitted

The second largest cause of reported medication incidents, according to the NPSA report (2007), is omitted medicines. The report highlighted serious and fatal outcomes for omissions of certain drugs such as anticonvulsants and insulin.

Recommendations for healthcare professionals.

- Do not ignore omissions caused by prescribing, dispensing or administering errors and report all serious omissions as a medication incident.

Recommendations for NHS organizations.

- Evaluate and audit all reports of omissions and delays. Results should be used to target areas of high reporting and to ensure systems are appropriate to reduce likelihood for the future.
- Review medicine storage and supply chains regularly.

Ensure the correct medicines are given to the correct patient

This section deals with two 'human error' categories:

- mis-selection of a drug
- mis-identification of a patient.

The NPSA is working with the pharmaceutical industry to improve medication package design and labelling to avoid confusion and mis-selection of drugs, which may occur at any time in the medication process.

Recommendations for healthcare professionals.

- Ensure awareness of drug names that look and sound alike. Colleagues should be alerted upon discovery of a drug that has a similar name to another.
- Store medicines that look or sound alike in different locations.
- Use labels that alert other users to the risk.
- Double check with a colleague before administration.
- Liaise with pharmacy department to use medicines with safer designs to minimize risk.
- For patients in hospital, avoid mis-identification of these patients by checking identification – using auto-ID technology (if available), hospital number, NHS number, date of birth and address where necessary.

Recommendations for NHS organizations.

- Be aware of the risks of medications that look and sound alike. Improve the medication system.
- Review reports of wrong medicine and wrong patient selection and identify medications most frequently mis-selected. Findings should be used to improve systems and minimize risk to patients.
- Improve and develop purchasing for safety policies and medicines.
- Ensure policies are in place for separate storage, alert labels and double checking to help minimize risk.
- Consider auto-ID technology.

Document patient's medicine allergy status

As a significant number of reported serious incidents involved patients who had a known allergy to medication, the NPSA has made the following recommendations.

Recommendations for healthcare professionals.

- Ensure medication allergy status is documented in patient's notes.
- Do not prescribe, dispense or administer a drug if you are unsure of the patient's allergy status.

Recommendations for NHS organizations.

- Audit the frequency of medication incidents involving patient allergy.
- Ensure all electronic prescribing and dispensing systems utilize a record of the patient's allergy status so that an alert is given prior to prescription or dispensing.
- For patients in hospital, use coloured wristbands for alerting staff to patients with known medication allergy.
- Ensure that systems are developed locally to ensure staff understand that some combinations of drugs may contain penicillin and could cause serious harm to patients with penicillin allergy (e.g. co-amoxiclav, co-fluampicil).

The NPSA also recommends that healthcare commissioners ensure that reporting and learning of medication incidents is a requirement for all commissioned services who are involved in the use of medicines.

All commissioned NHS organizations are also required to submit an Annual Report on their medication practice.

NPSA and NHS confederation in March 2008

Five key changes to improve patient safety by strengthening reporting and learning

In March 2008, the NPSA, together with an NHS confederation which consisted of 20 organizations with the highest reporting figures, shared their experiences and produced a briefing outlining five organizational changes to improve patient safety reporting.

The organization changes are briefly summarized below:

Change 1: Give feedback to staff.

It was felt that feedback on reporting was encouraging for staff and this motivated them to continue to report.

Methods of feedback included newsletters and case study reports among others.

Change 2: Focus on learning.

The focus of the 'blame culture' needs to shift so that the focus is more about what has been learned from incidents so that improvements may be made in that particular area to improve patient safety.

Change 3: Engage frontline staff.

There are suggestions about employing clinicians as 'safety champions' to flag up the issue at grass roots levels.

Change 4: Make it easy to report.

Access to forms needs to be easy with one well-designed form for all incidents. Organizations using web-based forms found improved consistency and efficiency in their reporting patterns.

Change 5: Make reporting matter.

It seemed that the organizations who robustly reported incidents had clear lines of strong leadership and their data were used to influence their decisions at a high level.

Summary

In conclusion, it has been well documented that medication errors are seriously under-reported and that the total number of reports has largely remained unchanged since the late 1980s. All healthcare professionals have a responsibility to report medication errors to help to reduce further recurrence. In order to improve reporting rates, there needs to be an increase in awareness of the need to report, together with standardized consistent education on the importance of pharmacovigilance as part of continuing professional development for all healthcare workers.

It is gratifying to see that, in recent years, the proportion of reports being submitted by nurses and pharmacists has increased (MHRA, 2008). With increased participation by other healthcare professionals in medications management and prescribing, perhaps it is now time for mandatory reporting of medication errors.

References

Audit Scotland (2008). A Scottish Prescription: managing the use of medicines in hospitals follow-up study. Project Brief (June 2008). http://www.audit-scotland.gov.uk/docs/fwd/pb_managing_medicines_followup.pdf

Barnes J, Anderson LA, Phillipson JD. (2003). Herbal Therapeutics. (10) Herbal Interactions. *Pharmaceutical Journal*, **270**(7233), 118–21.

Belton K, Lewis S, Payne S, Ralins MD, Wood SM. (1995). Attitudinal survey of adverse drug reaction reporting by medical practitioners in the United Kingdom. *British Journal of Clinical Pharmacology*, **39**, 223–6.

Bruce J, Wong I. (2001). Parenteral drug administration errors by nursing staff on an acute medical admissions ward during day duty. *Drug Safety*, **24**(11), 855–62.

Department of Health (2001). *National Service Framework for Older People*. London: Department of Health.

Elland I, Belton K, van Grootheest A, Meiners AP, Rawlins MD, Stricker BHCh. (1999). Attitudinal survey of voluntary reporting of adverse drug reactions. *British Journal of Clinical Pharmacology*, **48**(4), 623–7.

Ferner RE, Aronson JK. (2000). Medication errors, worse than a crime. *The Lancet*, **355**(9208), 947–8.

Hazell L, Shakir SA. (2006). Under reporting of adverse drug reactions: a systematic review. *Drug Safety*, **29**, 385–96.

Howard RL, Avery AJ, Slavenburg S, *et al.* (2007). Which drugs cause preventable admissions to hospital? A systematic review. *British Journal of Clinical Pharmacology*, **63**(2), 136–47.

MHRA website, Safety information: What to report, Causality. At www.mhra.gov.uk/home/idcplg?IdcService=SS_GET_PAGE&;nodeId=754 (accessed July 2008).

Morimoto T, Gandhi T, Seger A, Hsieh T, Bates D. (2004). Adverse drug events and medication errors: detection and classification methods. *Quality and Safety in Health Care*, **13**, 306–14.

National Patient Safety Agency (2004). *Seven Steps to Patient Safety*. London: NPSA.

National Patient Safety Agency (2007) *Safety in Doses: medication safety incidents in the NHS*. London: NPSA.

National Patient Safety Agency Briefing (2008). Act on reporting: five actions to improve patient safety reporting. Issue 161.

Pirmohamed M, James S, Meakin S, *et al.* (2004). Adverse drug reactions as cause of admission to hospital: prospective analysis of 18,820 patients. *British Medical Journal*, **329**, 15–19.

Sanders J, Esmail A. (2003). The frequency and nature of medical error in primary care: understanding the diversity across studies. *Family Practice*, **20**, 231–6.

World Health Organization (2005). *WHO draft guidelines for adverse event reporting and learning systems*. Geneva: WHO. http://www.who.int/patientsafety/events/05/Reporting_Guidelines.pdf

Williams DJP. (2007). Medication errors. *Journal of the Royal College of Physicians Edinburgh*, **37**, 343–6.

Ensuring safety through evidence-based medicine

Sharon Smart

Introduction

To offer our patients high quality and safe care, we must be prepared to base our decisions on the best available evidence, continually evaluate our own practice and seek to improve it, learn from unexpected incidents and errors (whether these are our own or others'), and share uncertainty with our patients and the NHS (to help prioritise the research agenda). In this chapter I outline the principles of evidence-based medicine, briefly mention some of its limitations and describe how it can help you practise safely. The chapter focuses on therapeutic interventions, but it is important to be aware that evidence-based medicine can support safe practice in other ways, for example, by informing you about the accuracy of diagnostic tests, the prognosis of a condition, and the causes and risk factors for a disease.

Evidence and evidence-based medicine

What is evidence?

In its broadest sense evidence is information that is used to support the truth of a recommendation or conclusion. Evidence is found in a wide variety of sources such as published research, expert opinion, patient experience and audit data.

What is evidence-based medicine?

Evidence-based medicine has been defined as the integration of best research evidence with our clinical expertise and our patient's unique values and circumstances (Straus *et al.*, 2000). The practice of evidence-based medicine requires the following steps (Dawes, 2005):

1. translation of uncertainty to an answerable question;
2. systematic retrieval of the best evidence available;
3. critical appraisal of evidence for validity, clinical relevance, and applicability;
4. application of results into practice;
5. evaluation of performance.

By putting these processes into practice you can help ensure the safety of your patients.

Medication Safety: An Essential Guide, ed. Molly Courtenay and Matt Griffiths. Published by Cambridge University Press. © M. Courtenay and M. Griffiths 2009.

Research evidence

How are evidence resources classified?

Brian Haynes suggested that evidence resources could be classified in a hierarchy (the 4S pyramid) (Haynes, 2001). His model can be adapted to include five categories, with studies at the base, syntheses (systematic reviews) the next level up, synopses of studies the level above this, summaries of the evidence and knowledge about a clinical topic above these, and evidence-based information systems at the top (see Fig. 11.1).

Studies

By studies we mean the reports of original research evidence that are published in journals and on-line. The different types of studies are described in Table 11.1.

Syntheses

By syntheses we mean systematic reviews. Systematic reviews use explicit methods to thoroughly search the literature, select all the relevant research, critically appraise the individual studies and use appropriate statistical techniques to combine the results in a meta-analysis.

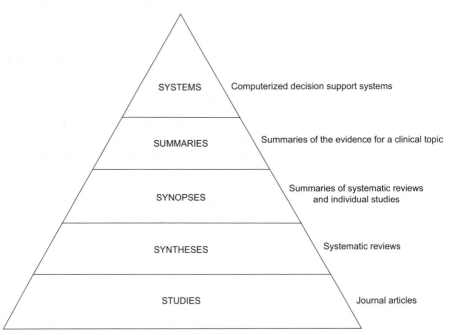

Figure 11.1. 5S classification of evidence resources.

Table 11.1. Types of studies

Classification	Study type	Description
Experimental	Randomized control trials	A group of patients is randomized into an experimental group and a control group. These groups are followed up for the variables/outcomes of interest.
Observational changes or differences in one characteristic (e.g. whether or not people received a specific treatment or intervention) are studied in relation to changes or differences in other(s) (e.g. whether or not they died), without the intervention of the investigator.	Cohort studies	Involves identification of two groups (cohorts) of patients, one that received the exposure of interest, and one that did not, and following these cohorts forward for the outcome of interest (prospective).
	Case-control	A study that involves identifying patients who have the outcome of interest (cases) and control patients who do not have that same outcome, and looking back to see if they had the exposure of interest (retrospective).
	Cross-sectional study	The observation of a defined population at a signal point in time or time interval. Exposure and outcome are determined simultaneously.
	Case series	A report on a series of patients with an outcome of interest. No control group is involved.
	Case report	A report on a single patient with an outcome of interest.
	Expert consensus	General agreement among experts following a decision-making process that seeks to resolve or mitigate objections.
	Expert opinion	The opinion of a group of experts.
	Qualitative studies	Studies that explore and understand people's beliefs, experiences, attitudes and behaviour through activities such as focus groups and in-depth interviews. They generate non-numerical data.

Synopses

By synopses we mean brief descriptions of the results of individual systematic reviews and studies. Synopses tend to focus on one aspect of research, e.g. a particular benefit or harm of an intervention.

Summaries

By summaries we mean distillations of all the relevant evidence about a clinical topic. They should help healthcare professionals decide what to do, when to do it and how to do it.

Systems

By systems we mean intelligent information systems or computerized decision support systems that link information in the electronic patient information to the best available knowledge about a clinical problem. These systems can be electronic guidelines, care pathways, or alerts and reminders. At present, such systems are not well developed or widely available.

What is the best research evidence?

By convention evidence has been assessed and ranked into hierarchies to reflect its validity or 'closeness to the truth'. Different hierarchies have been developed for different types of research questions to reflect the fact that different types of questions are better answered by different types of evidence. Even for questions about interventions, a number of hierarchies of evidence have been defined but the important thing to realize is that the type of evidence that is generally considered to be at the least risk of bias is at the top of the hierarchy and the type of evidence that is generally considered to be at the most risk of bias is at the bottom. In reality, there are limitations to the usefulness of this approach – the design of the study (type of research evidence) does not automatically reflect its quality, for example, systematic reviews with a high risk of bias may be no more valid than expert opinion.

What is the best research evidence for questions about the effectiveness of interventions (e.g. drugs)?

For questions about the effectiveness of interventions – RCTs are the study design of choice and systematic reviews of RCTs provide the highest level of evidence. If there are no RCTs available, look for non-randomized trials and cohort studies and case-control studies, and then finally look for case series or reports, expert consensus and expert reviews (opinion) in that order.

What is the best research evidence for questions about the harm of interventions?

For questions about the harms of interventions – look at RCTs *and* reports based on pharmacovigilance, e.g. Drug Safety Updates from the Medicines and Healthcare products Regulatory Agency *and* cohort studies and case-control studies. If these are not available, look for case series and reports.

What is a pragmatic approach to finding the best research evidence?

Sources of high-quality guidance in which recommendations have been formulated from summaries, synopses and syntheses of appraised evidence are a good place to start. If evidence-based guidance is not available, then follow the 5S principle: search information services that provide summaries of the evidence, and if that is unsuccessful search services that provide synopses, and if that doesn't yield anything search for syntheses, and then, as a last resort, look for individual studies.

It is worth remembering that pre-appraised sources should be considered before diving into the medical and nursing databases yourself. Finding, appraising and synthesizing the best primary research evidence can be a minefield – there is good evidence that journals are more likely to publish articles with positive findings (positive publication bias), that some abstracts emphasize the positive results within studies, that harms are less well presented than benefits, and that peer reviewers and editors fail to spot methodological and statistical mistakes within the articles.

This pragmatic approach is essential if you simply do not have the time or the experience to find, appraise and synthesize the best available evidence. Listed below are a number of high-quality, freely available resources provided to NHS healthcare professionals to enable them to practise safely in an evidence-based way. There are also high-quality resources available on a subscription basis, e.g. *Clinical Evidence and Drugs and Therapeutic Bulletin*.

Guidance

The National Institute for Health and Clinical Excellence provides national guidance on promoting good health and preventing and treating ill health for England and Wales (www.nice.org.uk).

The NHS Clinical Knowledge Summaries service (CKS) is a source of evidence-based guidance and practical 'knowhow' about the common conditions managed in primary care. It provides quick answers to clinical questions that arise in the consultation, linking to detailed answers that clearly outline the evidence on which they are based (www.cks.library.nhs.uk).

The Scottish Intercollegiate Guideline Network provides national clinical guidelines for Scotland (www.sign.ac.uk).

Summaries

The NHS Clinical Knowledge Summaries service (CKS) in addition to guidance, provides stand-alone evidence summaries. Through CKS, you can also access DynaMed, a clinical reference tool that provides evidence summaries on 3000 topics (www.cks.library.nhs.uk).

MeReC provides concise, evidence-based information about medicines and prescribing-related issues (www.npc.co.uk/merec.htm).

Synopses

Bandolier is a website about the use of evidence in health, healthcare and medicine (www.jr2.ox.ac.uk/bandolier).

The National electronic Library for Medicines provides timely and relevant information on medicines to support prescribing at the point of care (www.nelm.nhs.uk).

The Database of Abstracts of Reviews of Effectiveness (DARE) contains summaries of systematic reviews which have met strict quality criteria. Included reviews are about the effects of interventions. Each summary also provides a critical commentary on the quality of the review (www.york.ac.uk/inst/crd/crddatabases.htm#DARE).

The NHS Economic Evaluation Database (NHS EED) is designed to serve the needs of NHS decision-makers, and it can also be used as a research tool because it contains a pool of readily accessible critically appraised information (www.york.ac.uk/inst/crd/crddatabases.htm#NHSEED).

Syntheses

Cochrane Reviews are based on the best available information about healthcare interventions. They explore the evidence for and against the effectiveness and appropriateness of treatments (medications, surgery, education, etc) in specific circumstances. The complete reviews are published in The Cochrane Library (www.cochrane.org/reviews/).

The NIHR Health Technology Programme provides independent research information about the effectiveness, costs and broader impact of healthcare treatments and tests for those who plan, provide or receive care in the NHS (www.ncchta.org/project/htapubs.asp).

The Health Technology Assessment Database (HTA) contains information on healthcare technology assessments (www.york.ac.uk/inst/crd/crddatabases.htm#HTA).

How do you find studies?

There will be times where you will not be able to find evidence-based guidance, evidence summaries, or evidence synopses and you may wish to look for individual studies. The first step is to convert the need for information into an answerable question.

Formulating a question

Formulating the information you require into one or more structured questions makes it easier to find an answer from the large volume of medical literature that is available today. Most questions can be structured using a method known as PICO.

- Population and clinical outcome.
- Intervention (or indicator for an exposure to an environmental factor/physical feature, or index test for a diagnostic test).
- Comparator, i.e. what you are comparing the intervention/exposure/physical factor/test you are interested in with.
- Outcome, i.e. what you and/or the patient are interested in happening.

Sometimes a timeframe (T) is also added to the structured question (PICOT).

Imagine the following scenario. A 20-year-old woman comes to see you with weakness on the right-side of her face and difficulty closing her right eye. You make a diagnosis of Bell's palsy. Recently, a colleague told you that antiviral drugs can improve recovery and you want to know whether to prescribe these for your patient.

You can formulate this question as:

P = people with Bell's palsy;
I = antiviral drugs;
C = no antiviral drugs;
O = recovery.

Developing search terms

The next step is to use your PICO(T) question to develop terms to search with. You can do this by using the actual question terms, together with synonyms and alternative spellings.

The search terms you could use for the question above include Bell's palsy, Bell palsy, idiopathic facial nerve paralysis, antiviral, acyclovir, aciclovir, famciclovir, famcyclovir, valaciclovir, valacycolvir, recovery.

Where to search

MEDLINE® (Medical Literature Analysis and Retrieval System Online) is the US National Library of Medicine's® (NLM) bibliographic database that contains over 17 million references to journal articles in life sciences with a concentration on biomedicine.

- PubMed, a service of the National Library of Medicine, provides free internet access to Medline and other life science journals for biomedical articles back to the 1950s.
- NHS Evidence Health Information Resources (formerly the National Library for Health) provides free internet access to Medline for people with an NHS Athens password.
- Your local medical library.

Embase is a bibliographic database with over 11 million references of pharmacological and biomedical literature dating back to 1974.

- It can be accessed free through NHS Evidence Health Information Resources (formerly the National Library for Health) with an NHS Athens password.

CINAHL® is a bibliographic database with 5.5 million references to nursing, allied health literature and health sciences librarianship journal articles dating back from 1982.

- It can be accessed free through NHS Evidence Health Information Resources (formerly the National Library for Health) with an NHS Athens password.

Finding guidance and the best research evidence: NHS Evidence

Established by NICE and launched in April 2009, NHS Evidence is a web-based service that aims to help healthcare professionals find, access and use high quality clinical and non-clinical information, and best practice (www.evidence.nhs.uk). NHS Evidence consolidates information from a wide variety of sources and aims to become the 'first point of contact' for NHS staff looking for national, international and local evidence and related information.

Through NHS Evidence Health Information Resources (www.library.nhs.uk), you can access evidence-based reviews (including systematic reviews from the Cochrane Library), guidance (including the Clinical Knowledge Summaries and guidance from the National Institute for Health and Clinical Excellence), full text e-books and e-journals, patient information and drug information. You can also search PubMed and each of the following databases:

- Medline
- Embase
- Cinahl
- British Nursing Index
- PsycInfo (literature on psychology and allied health fields)
- AMED (information on complimentary/alternative medicine and palliative care)
- HMIC: Kings Fund and Department of Health data (information on healthcare management and policy).

Full texts of articles, purchased by the NHS, are available within the search interface next to the reference. You will need an NHS Athens password to access some of the content of NHS Evidence Health Information Resources (formerly the National Library for Health) (www.library.nhs.uk). Staff working for, or delivering services on behalf of, or in conjunction with, the NHS are eligible for an NHS Athens password.

How do I determine if the results of the study are likely to be 'true' or have been influenced by bias?

Whether you have searched for a piece of research to answer a clinical question or whether a new study has been published and you want to decide whether it will change your practice, the ability to understand if a piece of research is addressing the same or a sufficiently similar question to yours, how well a study was carried out to prevent the results from being affected by bias, and understanding what the results mean is a very valuable skill. It is beyond the scope of this book to describe how to critically appraise a piece of research in detail and if you wish to develop your critical appraisal skills there are many excellent evidence-based medicine courses, internet resources, and books available to help you to do so.

There are, however, some important concepts to be aware of.

- *Bias* – is *systematic* error that produces over- or under-estimation of a result or measurement. There are many different kinds of bias, and it is convenient to consider these in two categories:
  - Methodological bias. Bias arising from flaws in research methodology.
  - Framing bias. Bias arising from the way in which research results are presented and interpreted. Spin is framing bias, done with the intention to mislead.
- *Random allocation* to treatment groups (randomization) eliminates selection bias. Inadequate methods of treatment allocation can exaggerate the results (odds ratios) by more than 40% (Schulz, 1995).
- *Blinding* reduces reporting and observer bias. Single-blinded trials are ones in which either the subject or the observer are unaware of which treatment the subject has been given. Double-blinded trials are ones in which neither the subject nor the observer know which treatment has been given. Trials that are not double-blinded can exaggerate the results (odds ratios) by 17% (Schulz, 1995).
- *Confounding factors* are variables, other than the ones being measured in the study, which can affect the results of a study. If confounding factors are not measured and considered, they can result in bias.
- *Size of the clinical trial* – clinical trials should be designed using a power calculation to determine how many subjects need to be recruited to the trial to determine whether there is a difference between treatments (intervention and placebo or comparative treatment). The smaller the event rate being measured the more people will be required to be included in the study to demonstrate a difference.
- The *placebo effect* is the effect that is attributable to the *expectation* that a treatment will have an effect. If an intervention is compared to no treatment, the observed effect may be entirely due to the placebo effect. Ideally, an intervention should be compared to a placebo that is indistinguishable from the intervention to know if the intervention has an actual effect.
- *Sub-group analysis* is often carried out in studies to see if there are subgroups of trial subjects who are more (or less) likely to be helped (or harmed) by the intervention under investigation. Multiple comparisons between different subgroups will show an erroneous statistical difference between sub-group categories 5 times out of a hundred (when testing at the 5% level of significance) that has occurred because of chance. You should be suspicious of retrospective (not documented in the study's protocol) sub-group analysis and in general regard it as useful information to generate hypotheses for further testing, rather than evidence to change practice.

How are results in studies reported and what do they mean?

Results from analytical studies (RCTs, cohort studies, case-control studies) are presented as continuous or dichotomous data. Continuous data are data from outcomes that are measured on a continuous scale (e.g. blood pressure, pain). Dichotomous data are data from 'yes or no' outcomes where subjects must be in one or two groups (e.g. dead or alive, stroke or no stroke). The two outcome groups usually describe a good event and a bad event. Sometimes we see dichotomous data that has been made from data that was measured on a continuous scale, e.g. measurements of weight can be converted to overweight/obese and not overweight. The advantage of doing this is that it makes the data easier to analyse and, most importantly, easier to interpret. However, there are disadvantages to converting continuous data to dichotomous data; in particular, the size of the effect may be lost (someone may have lost weight when measured on a continuous scale but may not have lost enough weight to move from the overweight/obese group to the not overweight group).

Dichotomous data from subjects in a study are summarized in terms of risk, odds or numbers needed to treat to help us predict what will happen to others, i.e. our patients.

Risk and odds

Risk is the probability of having a specific event (either good or bad). It is calculated by dividing the number of people with the outcome by the total number of people who could have had the event. *Odds* is the risk of having an event (good or bad) divided by the risk of not having the event and can be calculated by dividing the number of events by the number of non-events.

Relative risk and odds ratio

We often want to know how effective an intervention is compared to no treatment or to other treatments that are commonly used and to help us understand this clinical trials provide the results as relative risk, odds ratios, relative risk reduction or absolute risk reduction.

Relative risk (RR) is the risk of the event in the experimental group divided by the risk of the event in the other group. It tells us how many times more likely the event will occur in the experimental group compared to the other group. Relative risk is a ratio and therefore a RR of 1 means that the experimental treatment had the same effect as the placebo or the comparative treatment. A RR of less than one means that the experimental treatment reduces the chance of the event, and a RR of more than one means that the experimental treatment increases the chance of the event (Table 11.2).

Table 11.2. What different levels of relative risk mean

Relative risk	What this means
Less than 1.0	The risk of harm/likelihood of benefit is reduced for the intervention compared to the control.
1.0	No increased or decreased risk for the intervention compared to the control.
1.0 – 2.0	The risk of harm/likelihood of benefit is higher for the intervention group compared to the control group, but most events occur because of underlying factors rather than the intervention.
More than 2.0	The risk of harm/likelihood of benefit is higher for the intervention group compared to the control group, but most events occur because of the intervention.

(Bandolier, 2007)

The odds ratio (OR) is the odds of the event occurring in the experimental group compared to the odds of the event occurring in the other group. Similar to relative risk an OR of 1 means that the experimental treatment had the same effect as the placebo or comparative treatment. An OR of less than one means that the experimental treatment reduces the chance of the event and an OR of more than one means that the experimental treatment increases the chance of the event.

When event rates are low (e.g. 1%) the OR is a close approximation of the RR; however, as the event rates increase this approximation becomes unacceptable and it can be misleading to interpret ORs as RRs.

Absolute risk difference

The absolute risk difference describes the absolute change in risk that is attributed to the experimental treatment. It is the risk of the event (good or bad) in the experimental group minus the risk of the event in the other group. If the absolute risk difference is 0, then the experimental treatment has the same effect as the placebo or the comparative treatment. If the absolute risk difference is less than 1, then the experimental treatment reduces the risk of the event (good or bad), and if the absolute risk difference is more than 1, then the experimental treatment increases the risk of the event. The absolute risk difference cannot be more than +1 or less than –1. As the absolute risk difference can be a small number and difficult to interpret, we sometimes see the absolute risk difference multiplied by 100 and described as a percentage reduction or increase in the event rate (e.g. an absolute risk difference of –0.01could be expressed as a 1% reduction in the event rate).

Relative risk reduction

Relative risk reduction is a commonly reported outcome measure and is the reduction in the event rate of the experimental group compared to the event rate in the other group.

Numbers needed to treat and numbers needed to harm

Perhaps the most user-friendly way of presenting (dichotomous) data from clinical trials to non-statisticians is the Number Needed to Treat (NNT). The NNT tells us the number of people we need to treat in order to prevent one bad event and should be linked to a time frame, e.g. we would need to treat three people *for 1 year* to prevent one death. It is the inverse of the absolute risk difference (with the minus sign dropped) and is usually rounded up to the next whole number. A very small NNT (i.e. close to 1) means that the intervention will be effective in nearly every person that receives it, and is quite unusual to find. A NNT of 2–3 indicates that the intervention is quite effective but even interventions with NNTs of up to 40 may still be considered clinically effective (McQuay and Moore, 1997). If you wish to compare the clinical effectiveness of a number of interventions for a condition, NNTs can be very helpful, so long as the *same* outcomes have been measured for each intervention and in similar populations. It is, however, inappropriate to compare the NNTs of interventions for different diseases, or when the populations differ with respect to their chances of responding to the intervention.

Occasionally, the Number Needed to Harm (NNH) is also reported. The NNH tells us the number of people who need to be exposed to the intervention or risk factor to cause harm in one person.

How certain can I be that the outcome(s) reported by the research evidence are NOT due to chance?

To understand if the results of the clinical trial were due to chance or to the effectiveness of the intervention we can look at the P-value and the confidence intervals (CIs).

The P-value measures the probability that a result is due to chance. A low P-value (usually 0.05 or less) means that the probability of the result being due to chance is low (5% or less) and we can be reasonably certain that the effect of the intervention is real. A P-value of 0.05 or less is often termed statistically significant.

It is possible that the calculated effect of treatment from a sample of the population (i.e. the subjects in a clinical trial) is an over- or under-estimation of the treatment effect that we would see if we treated the whole population (the real effect of treatment). Confidence intervals provide a range of values above and below the calculated effect of the treatment within which we can be reasonably sure that the real effect lies. You will usually see 95% CI, which means that there is a 95% chance that the range of values contains the real treatment effect. If the 95% CI for the difference between the experimental and the control group do not include 0 for a difference, or 1 for a ratio, then we can be reasonably confident that the result is not due to chance.

Limitations of the available research evidence

Length of follow-up in clinical trials

Even well-conducted clinical trials with a low risk of bias have limitations. Often, the follow-up of subjects is limited and the long-term impact of the intervention (both in terms of harm and benefit) is unknown. This is why post-licensing pharmacovigilance is so important.

Selective publishing

It is appropriate for the peer-review process to exclude reports of poorly conducted research evidence from publication. However, inappropriate publication bias is a common problem. Studies with a positive outcome are more likely to be published than studies with a negative outcome and are more likely to be published in journals with higher impact. Conclusions based exclusively on published studies are therefore likely to exaggerate the benefits of an intervention.

Groups commonly under-represented or excluded from clinical trials

Many studies do not include young and pregnant people.

Because of a lack of research evidence to license many of the drugs, prescribing for children is a particular problem with over a third of all prescriptions being prescribed outside of the product license (off label) (Conroy, 2000). To help address this issue, the

British National Formulary for Children (BNFC) provides information based on the best available evidence to support safe and effective prescribing for children of all ages from neonates to adolescents.

Most drugs also remain unlicensed for use in pregnancy because of a lack of research evidence about their effectiveness and safety. Some drugs have a long history of use in pregnancy without harming the fetus or mother and are considered safe to use. The National Teratology Information Service answers enquiries from NHS healthcare professionals about the toxicity of drugs and chemicals during pregnancy and can be contacted during office hours on 0191 260 6181. The service also collects data on specific drugs (and other hazards) that can be used to answer enquiries on the safety of drugs in pregnancy and to generate hypotheses that can be tested in epidemiological studies. Summaries of drug and chemical safety in pregnancy are available through the TOX-BASE website (www.spib.axl.co.uk).

Older people are often under-represented in studies and, as a consequence, we are often uncertain about the benefits and harms of interventions in this group. They are at greater risk of drug interactions as they are more likely to be taking more than one drug, metabolize and excrete drugs more slowly and are more likely to have co-existing disease than younger people.

Presentation of outcomes

Reports of research evidence often focus on the difference in outcomes between two or more groups, e.g. the difference between an intervention compared to a placebo, or the difference between two drugs. As described earlier, this difference can be described as an absolute difference or a relative difference. It is important to distinguish between the two when looking at the outcomes of a study, as which one is used will influence how big the difference seems. Relative differences are often more impressive than absolute differences, and the lower the baseline risk of an event, the larger the difference will be.

An example of this is the difference in the risk of developing a deep vein thrombosis in women taking different combined oral contraceptive pills. The World Health Organization Collaborative Study of Cardiovascular Disease and Steroid Hormone Contraception reported that the risk of deep vein thrombosis in women taking third-generation oral contraceptive pills (i.e. those containing the progestogens gestodene and desogestrel) was 2.6 times higher than for women taking older oral contraceptive pills (containing levonorgestrel) (WHO, 1995). However, it is important to consider this in the context of the absolute risk of women taking these pills developing a deep vein thrombosis, which is low – 15 per 100 000 women years for the second-generation pills and 25 per 100 000 women years for the third-generation pills (FFPRHC, 2007). The absolute risk difference is 10 per 100 000 women years or 0.0001. In other words, you would have to treat 10 000 women for a year with a third-generation pill rather than a second-generation pill to see one additional deep vein thrombosis.

Limited evidence for harm

The quality and quantity of reporting of harms in RCTs (regarded as the gold standard for evaluating the efficacy of interventions) are often inadequate and the trials are often not continued for long enough to find delayed harmful effects. In addition, the sample size of RCTs is often not big enough to detect rare adverse outcomes and to power the trials to do so is simply impractical. An analysis of over 1000 systematic reviews of healthcare interventions found that just over a quarter (27%) reviewed data on harm and only 4% focused primarily on safety (Chou and Helfand, 2005).

Is a cautious approach to adopting new research evidence good or bad?

There is evidence that the outcomes of single trials, however impressive the trials seem, should be interpreted with caution (Ioannidis, 2005). It is not unusual for subsequent studies to contradict the findings or to suggest the initial findings were exaggerated. This is particularly the case for non-randomized studies and for small randomized studies.

For example, the Nurses Health Study, a large prospective cohort study, found a reduction in the incidence of coronary artery disease and a reduction in death for cardiovascular disease in women receiving hormone replacement therapy (HRT), suggesting that HRT might have a cardio-protective effect in post-menopausal women (Stampfer *et al.*, 1991). However, subsequent RCTs have contradicted these findings. The HER and HER II studies showed no statistically significant reduction in coronary heart disease events in post-menopausal women with coronary heart disease (Hulley *et al.*, 1998; Grady *et al.*, 2002). The Women's Health Initiative showed that HRT increases the risk of coronary heart disease in women who start HRT more than 10 years after the menopause, but has not been shown to confer any statistically significant benefit for women who start HRT earlier (Rossouw *et al.*, 2002, 2007). It is now clear that HRT should not be prescribed for either the primary or secondary prevention of coronary heart disease.

Clinical expertise

It is important to remember that, although the research evidence will show that *on average* an intervention is effective, or that *on average* one intervention is more effective than another, this does not mean that this intervention is best for all individuals. Having found and understood the best available evidence for your clinical question, you now need to determine factors for *your particular patient*.

- Does the recommendation or evidence you have found apply to your patient?
- Can you translate the evidence you have found into a practical action?
- Have you balanced the benefits of an intervention with the risk of harm?
- Is it sensible for you to provide this intervention or test?

Does the recommendation or evidence you have found apply to your patient?

You need to ensure that the guidance you have identified is applicable to your patient, or that the subjects in the studies that you have identified are sufficiently similar to your patient – if they are not, the results of the study may not apply to your patient. In particular, look out for age, sex, and the presence or absence of comorbidities. Too often, you

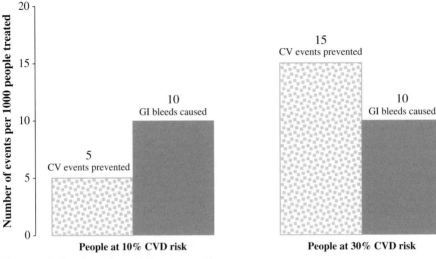

Figure 11.2. Benefits and harms of low dose aspirin treatment.

will see that the study population is older, younger or healthier than the typical patients that you are managing on a day-to-day basis.

Can you translate the evidence you have found into a practical action?

Things to consider include the following:

- Is the treatment available through the NHS?
- Is the intervention or test available in your area?

Have you balanced the benefits of an intervention with the risk of harm?

Harms from interventions include adverse drug effects, complications following surgery and emotional distress from psychological therapies. As outlined above, for most interventions, the body of evidence for harm is much less than for benefit and this increases the risk of coming to biased conclusions about the balance of benefit and harm. It is also important to consider the seriousness and reversibility of the harm as well as its frequency.

It is worth noting that, in general, the higher the risk that a patient has for an event (e.g. a myocardial infarction) before starting treatment the greater the absolute benefits of treatment will be. Conversely, patients at lower risk will experience less benefit.

Ideally, to balance benefits and harms you need to *quantify* the benefit and harms your particular patient is likely to experience. For most healthcare professionals, this is both difficult to do (because of the way trial data are presented) and impractical (because of the time that it takes to do). Using evidence-based guidance that reflects the association between degree of benefit and level of risk is much more practical!

To illustrate this point, consider the use of aspirin for the prevention of cardiovascular events. Aspirin treatment for 2 years has been shown to reduce cardiovascular events (non-fatal myocardial infarction, non-fatal stroke or vascular deaths) by 25% compared with placebo (Antithrombotic Trialists' Collaboration, 2002). Jane is a 55-year-old lady, whom you have estimated to have a 10% risk of developing cardiovascular disease over the next 10 years. Mary is a 55-year-old lady who you have estimated to have a 30% risk of having a cardiovascular event over the next 10 years. Without treatment, Jane has a 2 in 100 chance of having a cardiovascular event in the next 2 years and, with treatment, she has a 1.5 in 100 chance. Without treatment, Mary has a 6 in a hundred chance of having a cardiovascular event over the next 2 years and, with treatment, she has a 4.5 in 100 chance. The same meta-analysis quantified the risk of gastro-intestinal bleeding as 0%–2% over 52 months. This equates to a level of risk of up to 1% over 2 years for both Jane and Mary. Jane therefore will experience a small benefit from taking aspirin (an absolute risk reduction of 0.5% over 2 years), but this will be offset by the increased risk of gastro-intestinal bleeding (absolute risk increase of 0%–1% over 2 years), whereas the benefit that Mary will experience taking aspirin (absolute risk reduction of 1.5% over 2 years) is greater than the increased risk of gastrointestinal bleeding (absolute risk increase of 0%–1% over 2 years). In other words you have to treat 200 people like Jane, and 70 people like Mary, with aspirin for 2 years to prevent one cardiovascular event, with the expectation that one in every 100 people you treat will experience a gastro-intestinal bleed. It is important to note that the aspirin studies were carried out before it became best practice to prescribe prophylactic proton pump inhibitors for people at high risk of gastro-intestinal bleeding – and an estimate of the risk of harm consequently is lower (Fig.11.2).

Is it sensible for you to provide this intervention or test?

There are many things potentially to consider:

- If the intervention is a drug, is it licensed for this indication? – if not, do you feel competent to prescribe it?
- Do you have the resources to follow up and monitor the patient adequately?

Patient values

Evidence-based medicine is defined as the integration of best research evidence with clinical expertise and *patient values*. It is therefore important to ask your patient about his/her preferences, concerns and expectations about any proposed interventions or tests rather make a judgement as to what is in their best interest. The challenge is to translate the benefits of treatment and the risks of harm in a meaningful way to your patients. Patient decision aids are tools to help individuals become more involved in decision making by providing information about the options and outcomes and by clarifying personal values. They are appropriate to use when patients need to deliberate carefully about the personal value of the benefits and harms of options and are designed to complement, rather than to replace, discussion with a healthcare professional. There is evidence that decision aids work in that they reduce the proportion of patients who are uncertain what to do, increase participation in decision making without increasing anxiety and create realistic personal expectations of outcomes (O' Connor *et al.*, 1999). However, the impact of decision aids on satisfaction with decision making is uncertain.

To date, validated decision aids have not been widely deployed, but with an increasing emphasis on shared decision making they may be valuable tools for the future.

Highlighting uncertainty and feeding this into the research agenda

There are a number of initiatives to guide the research community to provide the research evidence that healthcare professionals and patients need to make decisions about healthcare. These include the following:

- The NICE research and development programme aims to promote research and development to improve patient care, particularly in areas where better evidence has the potential to radically improve care. Part of the process of developing NICE guidance is to identify gaps in the research evidence and to describe them as research recommendations. A key role of the NICE research and development programme is to prioritize, clearly present and effectively communicate these recommendations to the research community.
- The Database of Uncertainties about the Effects of Treatments is an on-line database that records uncertainties about the effects of treatments and draws on patients', carers' and clinicians' questions about the effects of treatments, research recommendations in reports of systematic reviews and clinical guidelines, and ongoing research. It is being developed to help those prioritizing research in the UK to take account of the information needs of patients, carers and clinicians. For more information, go to www.duets.nhs.uk.

Learning from mistakes and surprises is also EBM

Reports of medical errors and unexpected incidents that are not indexed in Medline will not be found in a conventional search of the medical literature. They do, however, provide us with evidence on which we can base safe clinical practice.

- The National Reporting and Learning System (NRLS), set up by the National Patient Safety Agency, collects reports of patient safety incidents from NHS organizations in England and Wales; analyses the data and reports the statistics to the NHS and the public; and provides alerts, directives and guidance, which can be locally implemented to strengthen the culture of patient safety.
- Confidential Enquiries into suicide and homicide, maternal and child health and patient outcome and death are commissioned and monitored by the NPSA.
- The Yellow Card scheme operated by the Medicines and Healthcare Regulatory Agency (MHRA) and the Commission on Human Medicines (CHM) acts as an early warning system for previously unrecognized reactions to drugs. An electronic bulletin containing the latest clinical information and clinical advice is published each month.

Supporting evidence-based practice in the future

Despite the ever-increasing volume of evidence on which we can base our clinical decisions and the development of clinical guidelines that interpret and apply that evidence, the healthcare provided by clinicians too often falls short of optimum. One solution to address the problem of implementing evidence-based medicine is the development of information systems that provide patient-specific assessments and/or recommendations to improve decision making – computerized decision support systems. Such systems have been developed to support the making of a diagnosis, to alert the healthcare professionals to abnormal values, as reminders for preventative health tasks, to provide advice for prescribing, to critique healthcare ordering and to provide evidence-based suggestions for patient management. The systems can provide information in a variety of forms, ranging from relatively simple pop-up boxes to intelligent computerized care pathways.

Clinical decision support systems have been shown to improve clinical practice, but not universally (Garg *et al.*, 2005; Kawamoto *et al.*, 2005). For clinical decision support systems to improve clinical practice, they must minimize the time, effort and initiative that it takes a healthcare professional to be presented with, and act on, a recommendation. Features that are associated with successful decision support systems include:

- decision support provided automatically as part of workflow;
- decision support presented at the point of decision making;
- recommendations that are actionable;
- computer-based systems.

Despite the growing evidence to support the use of computerized decision support systems to improve the safety and quality of healthcare, uptake has been slow. With the widespread introduction of electronic health records and the improved performance and evaluations of such systems, I believe we will see greater deployment of these systems in the not-too-distant future.

Conclusion

Evidence-based medicine underpins safe practice by supporting you to make the right diagnosis, to consider the most appropriate and effective options for management, to balance the risks of harm against the potential for benefit of an intervention and to communicate these with your patient, and to follow up and monitor your patients. On its own, it can never *ensure* safety, but it can reduce the risk of you harming your patients.

However, it is unrealistic to expect busy healthcare professionals to integrate best research evidence with clinical expertise and patient values and circumstances for all the decisions they have to make without the practical tools to do so. Studies and systematic reviews simply take too long to read, to appraise, to interpret and to implement. Synopses and summaries of the evidence, although quick to read, are often not orientated to the problems seen in day-to-day practice and are therefore difficult to implement. Problem-orientated, high-quality guidance is the best tool we have at present to support busy healthcare professionals to practice in a safe and evidence-based way. Increasingly, we will see such guidance implemented in user-friendly intelligent systems as alerts, reminders, prompts and electronic care pathways.

References

Antithrombotic Trialists' Collaboration (2002). Collaborative meta-analysis of randomised trials of antiplatelet therapy for the prevention of death, myocardial infarction and death in high risk patients. *British Medical Journal*, **324**, 71–86.

Bandolier (2007). On limitations. Bandolier. www.jr2.ox.ac.uk/bandolier/band161/b161-2.html [Accessed 29.04.08].

Chou R, Helfand M. (2005). Challenges in systematic reviews that assess treatment harms. *Annals of Internal Medicine*, **142**, 1090–9.

Conroy S, Choonara I, Impicciatore P, *et al.*, (2000). Survey of unlicensed and off label drug use in paediatric wards in European countries. *British Medical Journal*, **320**, 79–82.

Dawes M, Summerskill W, Glasziou P, *et al.*, (2005). Sicily statement on evidence-based practice. *BMC Medical Education*, 5:(1), www.biomedcentral.com/1472–6920/5/1.

FFPRHC (2007). First Prescription of Combined Oral Contraception. *Faculty of Family Planning & Reproductive Health Care*, www.ffprhc.org.uk/admin/uploads/FirstPrescCombOralContJan06.pdf [Accessed 29.04.08].

Garg AX, Adhikari NKJ, McDonald H, *et al.* (2005). Effects of computerized clinical decision support systems on practitioner performance and patient outcomes. *Journal of the American Medical Association*, **293**, 1223–38.

Grady D, Herrington D, Bittner V, *et al.*, HERS Research Group (2002). Cardiovascular outcomes during 6.8 years of hormone therapy: Heart and Estrogen/progestin Replacement Study follow-up (HERS II). *Journal of the American Medical Association*, **288**, 49–57.

Haynes RB. (2001). Of studies, syntheses, synopses and systems: the '4S' evolution of services for finding current best evidence. *Evidence Based Medicine*, **6**, 36–8.

Hulley S, Grady D, Bush T, Herrington D, Riggs B, Vittinghoff E. (1998). Randomized trial of estrogen plus progestin for secondary prevention of coronary heart disease in postmenopausal women. Heart and Estrogen/progestin Replacement Study (HERS) Research Group. *Journal of the American Medical Association*, **280**, 605–13.

Ioannides JPA. (2005). Contradicted and initially stronger effects in highly cited clinical research. *Journal of the American Association*, **294**, 218–28.

Kawamoto K, Houlihan C, Balas EA, Lobach DF. (2005). Improving clinical practice using clinical decision support systems: a systematic review of trials to identify features critical to success. *British Medical Journal*, **330**, 765–8.

McQuay HJ, Moore RA. (1997). Using numerical results from systematic reviews in clinical practice. *Annals of Internal Medicine*, **126**, 712–20.

O'Connor AM, Rostom A, Fiest V, *et al.* (1999). Decision aids for patients facing health treatment or screening decisions: systematic review. *British Medical Journal*, **319**, 731–4.

Rossouw JE, Anderson GL, Prentice R, *et al.*, Writing Group for the Women's Health Initiative Investigators (2002). Risks and benefits of estrogen plus progestin in healthy postmenopausal women: principal results from the Women's Health Initiative randomized controlled trial. *Journal of the American Medical Association*, **288**, 321–33.

Rossouw JE, Prentice RL, Manson JE, *et al.* (2007). Postmenopausal hormone therapy and risk of cardiovascular disease by age and years since the menopause. *Journal of the American Medical Association*, **297**, 1465–77.

Schulz KF, Chalmers I, Hayes RJ, Altman DG. (1995). Empirical evidence of bias: dimensions of methodological quality associated with estimates of treatment effects in controlled trials. *Journal of the American Medical Association*, **273**, 408–12.

Stampfer MJ, Colditz GA, Willett WC, Manson JE, Rosner B, Hennekens CH. (1991). Postmenopausal oestrogen therapy and cardiovascular disease. Ten year follow-up from the nurses' health study. *New England Journal of Medicine*, **325**, 756–62.

Straus SE, Richardson WS, Glasziou P, Haynes RB. (2005). *Evidence-based Medicine: How to Practise and Teach EBM*, 3rd edition. Edinburgh: Elsevier Churchill Livingstone.

World Health Organization Collaborative Study of Cardiovascular Disease and Steroid Hormone Contraception (1995). Effect of different progestagens in low oestrogen oral contraceptives on venous thromboembolic disease. *Lancet*, **346**, 1582–8.

Index